T0248367

IN THESE
STREETS

IN THESE STREETS

STREETS

REPORTING FROM THE FRONT LINES OF
INNER-CITY GUN VIOLENCE

Josiah Bates

JOHNS HOPKINS UNIVERSITY PRESS | BALTIMORE

Johns Hopkins University Press
2715 North Charles Street
Baltimore, Maryland 21218
www.press.jhu.edu

Library of Congress Cataloging-in-Publication Data

Names: Bates, Josiah, 1993– author.
Title: In these streets : reporting from the front lines of inner-city gun violence /
    Josiah Bates.
Description: Baltimore : Johns Hopkins University Press, [2024] |
    Includes bibliographical references and index.
Identifiers: LCCN 2023037098 | ISBN 9781421448985 (hardcover) |
    ISBN 9781421448992 (ebook)
Subjects: LCSH: Firearms and crime—United States. | Gun control—United States. |
    United States—Social conditions.
Classification: LCC HV7436 .B384 2024 | DDC 363.330973—dc23/eng/20231127
LC record available at https://lccn.loc.gov/2023037098

A catalog record for this book is available from the British Library.

Special discounts are available for bulk purchases of this book. For more information,
please contact Special Sales at specialsales@jh.edu.

For Mom and Dad
I'm eternally grateful for all the sacrifices you've made for me

CONTENTS

PREFACE

Family Stories

I grew up in Brownsville, Brooklyn. It's a notorious neighborhood in New York City. People from the city who don't live there think it's a war zone. I'm from Brownsville, but I'm not from the streets of Brownsville. I was a stoop kid: much of my time was spent in and around the house. Along with my cousins—there were five of us—I'd play at a park across the street or in the backyard. We were always chasing each other and fighting. My great-grandparents had a house on a pretty tame block in the neighborhood, but all around us was the anguish that is Brownsville. Our block, though, felt like a real community. My mom and I initially lived there on our own while my father was living in the Bronx, about 20 miles away, before moving to Brooklyn. Though my parents weren't together when I was born, both of them raised me.

I was a shy kid and mostly kept to myself. If I wasn't around family or a few close friends, I didn't have much to say. That and the fact that I had parents who kept a close eye on me are what steered me away from the streets. But in my heart, I felt like I was missing something by not hanging out on the block. As a kid, I always looked up to my uncle Shaka Mandela (now legally Devon French). He's only a few years older than me and was like a big brother. Shaka had swagger and confidence. Everyone was drawn to him, and it felt like he knew everyone in the neighborhood. I wanted to be like him, but I was just too shy.

Shaka had this poise about him. The way he rapped along to music was cool. He would sit on the front porch with his friends and just talk; they'd laugh and make digs at each other. I'd eavesdrop. I never knew what he was talking about, but it sounded so much more interesting than the cartoons I was watching on television. Even the way his mother (my grandmother) called him back to the house was captivating. In the summer, when the sun was setting, she would stand on the front porch and go "psst" loudly a few times, assuming Shaka was in the area. When he heard that, he knew it was time to come back home.

Shaka and I moved in different circles. Unfortunately, though, if you're Black and grew up in an inner-city neighborhood in this country, it's virtually impossible not to be affected by the crime and gun violence that goes on, either directly or through your family and friends.

Shaka has plenty of stories from his time on the block or in the projects. He remembers the first time he almost got shot. When he was around 10 years old, he was walking to a Blockbuster Video store not far from where he was living at the time in Bedford-Stuyvesant. It must've been cold out, because he had on a big puffy jacket—the kind that screamed "street cred" in the late 1990s. As he walked, he heard three loud bangs in a row. He felt like they were going off beside him, right next to his ear. Almost instinctively, Shaka ducked. "I just positioned myself in between the cars, and wherever I assumed the shots were coming from, that's where I tried to avoid," Shaka says. The shots came from a car on the street; the shooter was targeting someone in another car. After it all settled down, Shaka rose, but his jacket got caught on one of the cars, which tore a hole in it. He says he wore that jacket every single day that winter and that the hole reminded him of his first experience with gun violence.

In the decades since, Shaka has been around "countless" shootings. He can't remember how many people he knows who have been shot and killed. "It's weird too because I'm kind of forgetful, and it's sad because I forgot a lot of these niggas' names," Shaka says. "I got friends that died 10 years ago; you know how much life I lived since they died?" Now he's pretty far removed from that environment, working as a wind technician in Rhode Island. He'll chuckle sometimes as he reminisces about some of these events, but he knows the impact they've had on him and his community. "When you take a drug and it has side effects, this is the side effect," Shaka says. "This is a side effect of no jobs, no education, no resources. When you're poor it's an us-against-them mentality."

Hearing these kinds of stories and witnessing the violence myself as I grew up would eventually inspire me when I pursued a career in journalism.

Fast-forward to February 2020. I was sitting at my desk in the *Time* magazine office right next to Bryant Park in New York City. By this point, *Time* employees based in the city had only been in the space for a few months; we were previously in the Meredith Building in Lower Manhattan. It was the nicest office space I ever worked in. But the funny thing is I actually preferred the setup of our new midtown office, which resembled a traditional newsroom. Every time I exited the elevators onto our floor, I felt like I was in the *Washington Post* newsroom from *All the President's Men*.

By February 2020 I had only been at *Time* for less than nine months and was still getting used to my job, but I loved every second of working there.

As I look back now, February 2020 is crucial to everything about this book. It was about a month before the COVID-19 pandemic would really begin in the United States and change the face of the country and the rest of the world. By this point, I was certainly aware that the coronavirus was starting to make global headlines, but like a lot of other people, I wasn't that concerned. I didn't believe that there was much to worry about. My attention was focused on my beat as a reporter, which was criminal justice issues, particularly gun violence.

At first, I had wanted to cover sports. Once I got to college, though, my attention shifted. My own personal experiences and those of my family made criminal justice issues more appealing for me as a journalist. When it came to gun violence, I didn't understand why no one in the mainstream media seemed to care about the hundreds of Black people who are killed every day in our communities. I wanted to give those stories the attention I felt they deserved. When I joined *Time* in June 2019, it was an honor to be able to cover them for such a legacy news outlet. I grew up hearing about gun violence and being around it; now I'm covering it as a journalist.

As 2019 was winding down, I was working on an end-of-year roundup about several cities that had experienced an uptick in gun violence incidents. I wanted it to run in January 2020, but there were a lot of discussions on the right time to publish the piece. In journalism, the timing of when certain stories are published depends on the news peg—a trending topic in the mainstream media that makes a specific story relevant. So if there's a nationwide food shortage that has the attention of politicians, media outlets will be eager to publish news stories about food shortages. Gun violence in the Black community is not that story. It's an age-old tale that doesn't move the needle in the eyes of many national newsroom decision-makers unless there's a white cop pulling the trigger. In my experience, stories about the Black community entail a higher burden of justification.

I was still working on this story in February 2020. I had a crucial interview to do one day. It was with a Johns Hopkins University professor named Daniel Webster, one of the leading experts on this issue. This was my first time speaking with him. I was trying to get some perspective from him on the state of gun violence in the country.

As we wrapped up the call, he made a comment about the concerns around the coronavirus and gun violence. He suggested that if there were a situation in which a virus like that spread and everything had to shut down to stop the spread, that could be a disaster for daily shooting incidents. Curious, I asked him to explain that a bit more. He said that if police, social services, and other types of programs that are used to combat inner-city shootings have to be suspended, it could have a negative impact. Essentially, if another public health crisis started while the country was trying to deal with the gun violence crisis, there would be problems. I took note of that comment and thanked him for his time. I had no idea how right he would be, or that a couple of years later I'd be writing a book about that very subject.

Gun violence touches so many lives in the country. It's unquantifiable how far-reaching the problem is. I decided to write this book at the end of 2020, after the country had experienced one of the most devastating years of gun violence ever recorded. All the numbers will be explained later, but it cannot be overstated how bad it was. Unfortunately, 2020 was not an anomaly; the problem would persist for years.

Gun violence doesn't just touch the people who are shot or the people who pull the trigger, or even the family members of both sides. At this point in America, we are all affected by gun violence in one way or another—the paramedic who responds to a gunshot victim, the surgeon who removes the bullet or declares the victim dead, the pastor who provides comfort for the grieving family, the teachers who try to protect their students from the despair of the inner city, the parents who worry about their children at school, the family whose loved one died by suicide. Even those of us who have never seen or held a gun in our lives are affected by the psychological toll of gun violence. We all worry about our loved ones and whether they will make it home from the grocery store, movie theater, concert, mall, or school.

In June 2022, when I was writing this preface, the country was a couple of weeks removed from two heartbreaking mass shootings that grabbed everyone's attention. A gunman armed with a semiautomatic rifle killed 10 people outside a supermarket in Buffalo, New York; and 21 people—19 elementary school students and 2 teachers—died in the Uvalde, Texas, school shooting. By early July 2022, however, over 18,000 people had already been killed as a result of shootings since January. Most of these deaths were driven by inner-city community gun violence and suicides.

In an average year, gun violence costs the United States $557 billion, according to a July 2022 report by Everytown for Gun Safety—the largest gun-violence prevention organization in the United States. That's just a snapshot of economic consequences. The nonstop cycle of gun violence has enormous emotional and psychological repercussions. I spent much of 2020 writing about this problem as a journalist, though there was no shortage of prominent news topics in 2020. The pandemic was in full swing, the murder of George Floyd had started one of the largest protest movements in history, and of course, it was a particularly divisive election year. While I understood the importance of those topics, my attention was on gun violence. But I wasn't just focusing on the problem. I paid a lot of attention to the solutions that community leaders, residents, activists, experts, law enforcement, and city leaders were demanding. I learned through all my reporting that there are tangible solutions to this problem. I wanted to make sure that my coverage highlighted those.

Even while I cover this topic, I'm shocked at how far reaching gun violence's effects can be. I always go back to my own family. My cousin Christian is a few years younger than me. He spent most of his life in Atlanta. He worked his way through college and is now a photographer, taking pictures of local athletes, musicians, concerts, and any event he can get paid for. His goal is to develop his photography business and work with more high-profile clients. Christian is a vibrant and loving young man. You'd know right away if you met him that he's not a gangster. It's all about family for him, but he's been through a lot. He's lost at least seven friends to gun violence. That doesn't include the people he knew but with whom he didn't have a relationship who were killed in his neighborhood.

"It just has you on edge all the time. I feel like I gotta pay extra attention when I'm outside. If paying attention can stop me from getting grazed by a bullet, then I'm cool with that," Christian says. "I can't prevent myself from dying from a shooting but I can do my best to protect myself." The first person he knew who was killed was the babysitter he had when he was 10 years old. This was also the first person he ever saw with a gun. The babysitter was planning a robbery.

The babysitter was killed as soon as he kicked in the door of the house he was breaking into. Christian was devastated when he heard about it. "I was with this man every day," Christian recalls. "When *Batman Begins* came out, me and him watched that on bootleg together. I remember just being scared after that. Thinking one day I was going to get shot too." Christian is desperate to get out of his environment, and the only thing keeping him in the neighborhood is his mother: he doesn't want to leave her there alone. "It's just too much, I seen too many people running from gunshots," he says. "Who wants to live like that?"

Timothy (Timmy) Roberts is another cousin. I've always looked up to Timmy like I've looked up to Shaka. By the time Timmy was 17 years old, he had so much responsibility in the family. He was working a full-time job and helped to support his mother. My father spoke and dealt with him like he was an adult even at such a young age. One night nearly 20 years ago, Timmy was hanging out with friends at a club in the Bronx when he was shot in the leg. He was just at the wrong place at the wrong time.

One night when I was a baby, my dad came to visit me in Brooklyn after work. He had to go back home to the Bronx afterward, which was on the other side of the city from where my mother and I lived. After a train ride that lasted over an hour, he was walking down the stairs of the station when two young men robbed him at gunpoint. My father is tall, around six feet four inches. He remembers how small the two were and how tiny the gun was. His pride kicked in for a minute. Getting robbed by two kids was a little embarrassing for him, but he knew it made no sense to fight. He gave them his wallet and kept moving. "Them little motherfuckas got me that night," he says. It's not that big of a deal to him now, but it could have gone a different way. I could have lost him right there.

Before I was born, my mother was at a bus stop with a friend when someone walked up, pointed a gun, and told them to give up what they had. She chuckles about it today because the robber took her little purse, which had nothing in it. "He must've looked at me and thought I had money or something," she says. She has a less comical memory of when she saw someone get shot three times. She heard an argument going on between two guys outside. When she peeked out the window to see, one of the guys pulled a gun out, and as the other ran he took three bullets to the back. She saw the man fall on the car right in front of the house.

My stepfather has had three experiences with gun violence. One of these took place in college at Norfolk State in Virginia in the early 1990s. He was riding in a car on his way back to his apartment from a basketball game with a couple of friends, when a car high-beamed them. It followed them to their apartment complex, but they didn't think much of it. Once they got out, someone from the other car started shooting at them. My stepfather took off. "It was the fastest I ever ran in my life," he recalls. He jumped over a fence and kept running. One of his friends caught up to him as well. It turned out to be a case of mistaken identity. My stepfather and his friends just happened to be riding around in a car that looked similar to someone else's.

When I was 12 years old, I was robbed at gunpoint a block away from my home in Brownsville after going to a nearby store. The interval between the moment when the guy pulled the gun out and the moment he walked away felt like it lasted for hours, though it was probably less than a minute. My family likes to make fun of me and say I was a crybaby as a kid, so I'm surprised that when this happened I didn't really show any emotion. I just froze. When I saw the gun pointed at my chest, I genuinely believed that my life was going to end that night. I just thought, "Welp, this is it." Fortunately, the gunman just took my phone and my wallet and ran off. To this day, I haven't told my mother about it. I knew if I had told her that night, it would have turned into a big deal, so I just tucked it away and moved on. As time went by, I stopped thinking it was that big a deal. I can't remember how many times I heard gunshots outside my window.

I bring up all these examples to paint a picture. These are the stories of just a few people from one family who all have their own experiences with gun violence spanning several decades, whether it's being victims themselves, knowing victims, almost being victims, or perpetrating the violence. While this issue affects all of us, it's primarily a burden for Black people in the hood. My family is just an everyday group of people. We're what you would call "decent people" trying to get by. We come from blue-collar Caribbean workers.

I know this will be hard for some people to read. It was hard for my editor to read. In one of our conversations, he was amazed at how "matter of fact" these stories about my family come across.

The truth is we all feel incredibly lucky because no one in our immediate family has been killed by a gun. This is not the case for a lot of Black families from the inner city. That's how bad this problem is. I've spoken with people who have lost everyone close to them because of countless senseless shootings in the hood. These are folks who get ignored by policymakers.

There are no quick fixes to gun violence. We've tried some before and they haven't worked. That's because gun violence is complex. When it comes to complex issues, I tend to look at them from a journalistic perspective. I want to understand all the details and nuances. This book is about those nuances. It's about the nuances of the issue and the nuances of the solutions. Neighborhood leaders, law enforcement officials, activists, experts, victims, and even those who have pulled the trigger on someone will have to be heard if we want to understand the problem. Those are the people I'm highlighting in this book. As requested by certain sources, I use pseudonyms for some people to protect their identities. Community violence is the driver of a lot of this, but we can't ignore other types of gun violence like domestic violence or suicide. Those are equally important and must be addressed as well. Gun violence, particularly community gun violence, is a public health crisis.

A public health crisis can be defined as a strenuous health issue that affects people in at least one geographic area. This kind of crisis tends to affect all facets of life in that area. COVID-19 is the perfect example. It just so happened that it touched almost every aspect of society. Gun violence does the same thing, but specifically for poor Black communities.

I'm not much of a political person; I have no allegiance to any political party. I only say that to stress that this is not about politics, at least not for the people who truly deal with gun violence. If you ask people on the streets who have to duck bullets to get home, they will say they couldn't care less about what side of the aisle someone is on. Some might feel like certain solutions laid out in this book lean too much on one side or the other; I don't care about that: Both parties have failed—from city governments all the way up to the federal level. They have failed to protect these communities from gun violence. They've failed the most marginalized and vulnerable people in our society. They've failed hardworking, decent people like my family. The solutions to this problem are comprehensive and require more than whatever hot talking point a given political party focuses on when gun violence is trendy to discuss. This is about the people who are harmed by the problem every day and how our country can stop ignoring them.

PART I

The Drastic Rise

1

A Surge like No Other

"I would describe our work as amazing, complicated, dangerous, and absolutely necessary," Roy Alfonso, late 40s, says. "It's more than a job; it's a life's mission." Roy is calm, laid back, and sturdy, and he carries a wealth of knowledge with him, not just about the streets but about life in general. When someone asks him a question, he takes a full second's pause to answer thoughtfully. When he talks, it's like he's reading an essay; he doesn't waste a word. When you speak with him, he looks you in the eye. He wants you to know you're being heard and that your time is not being wasted. "He's sincere, he has a kind spirit and truly cares about other people," one community member says of Roy. He's also a true streetwise New Yorker. Just a few words and you'll hear the accent of someone who's familiar with the block: "He ova there, ain't he?" But his work gives him a bit more of a professional vibe.

Years ago, when Roy decided to dedicate his life to combating gun violence, it was his opportunity to have a positive impact on his community. In his past life, he contributed to some of the despair, pain, and violence that existed in the Bedford-Stuyvesant, Brooklyn, neighborhood he grew up in. In his next role, as a healer, he focused on prevention, working as a violence interrupter.

Violence interruption is a community-based approach to addressing gun violence. An interrupter is typically someone who was previously very active in the streets and has a level of credibility when trying to resolve conflicts in the neighborhoods in which they operate. Violence interrupters do not work with the police, and they are not armed. They treat gun violence as a disease, something spreading in a community that needs to be addressed from a multitude of angles.

There are different types of mediation methods. If a shooting incident occurs in an area where they work, the violence interrupters will try to gather as much information as they can and work to stop any retaliation. If they know someone is about to go shoot someone else, they'll try to stop them. Sometimes after a shooting incident, they'll organize a larger community response in and around the spot where the shooting happened. Sometimes they'll host events that have nothing to do with violence, just to get the community together. It could be a basketball tournament, a barbecue, or a back-to-school supplies giveaway.

Historically, Bed-Stuy has struggled with crime and gun violence. During the crack epidemic of the 1980s, when Roy was growing up, it was one of the most volatile communities in all of New York City. During this period, the train stations in the neighborhood would be deserted out of fear. The motto "Do or die Bed-Stuy" came from this era. After his release from prison, where he had spent over 20 years educating and rehabilitating himself while incarcerated for armed robbery, Roy was an ideal person to resolve the conflicts in the hood. "I was part of the problem growing up, so to be able to try and make the community safer and healthier for others is a blessing," he says. When he was putting work in on the streets, you knew not to mess with him. Today, Roy does not have a hint of that in him.

In Bed-Stuy, buildings are pressed together, with no spaces between them other than the streets. They all have the same beige-

and-brown look. Most people rent. Graffiti, garbage cans, and dumpsters are spread about. On hot summer days, the stink of garbage blends with the aroma of grilled food or the scent of foliage from the trees. Cars occupy almost all the parking spaces, which is odd because it seems like everyone in this neighborhood walks or uses public transportation. You can walk to the corner store, the laundromat, and the subway station. It's not the open-air drug market it used to be in the '70s and '80s.

In the summer of 2017, Roy was with a colleague, Bobby, working in Bed-Stuy near the Louis Armstrong public housing complex. The 2017 Bed-Stuy is much different from what it was in the 1980s and '90s, though the architecture hasn't changed: brownstone homes, apartment buildings, and more projects. The "do or die" motto isn't heard as often because of the neighborhood's gentrification, though some of the roots can still be found. The Louis Armstrong projects aren't like other public housing buildings in the city that are nearly skyscrapers; they resemble the less intimidating residential buildings in the neighborhood. During the summer in New York City, the immediate area around housing projects can be lively. Roy recalls "people being flooded out there" on this particular day in 2017. Kids and adults alike were out and about.

Bobby was also a violence interrupter. He was mediating a conflict between two guys near a bus stop. The disagreement was over a pair of sneakers. One of the individuals was supposed to give the other money for the sneakers, but the money hadn't been paid. On the streets, a debt like this can be a death wish. Though he wasn't taking the lead on this particular mediation, Roy watched closely, serving as backup for his colleague in case the situation escalated. He stood cool and collected while Bobby did all the work. Before they got to the scene, Bobby told him this had the potential to get out of hand. The seller was very angry. But the intervention was going well. Bobby let the two men go back and forth with their points. The seller wanted the money immediately. The buyer said he only agreed to pay after he wore the shoes and made sure he liked them, and he hadn't worn them yet. Bobby convinced the buyer to come up with the money by the end of the week. Reflecting, Roy thinks it's funny that they needed someone to step in and reach that logical conclusion, but sometimes "it be like that," he says.

All of a sudden, Roy noticed some commotion down the block—loud noises and yelling that all drowned itself out, like a section of a restaurant with a large party. To Roy's ears, it sounded drastic and dramatic. The two ran over.

When they got there, they saw three guys beating up another one on the corner. Spectators watched, some egging it on while others just observed. Then you had the ones who just took a peek while walking by. Bobby's instincts were to immediately break it up, but Roy stopped him. "I was like, wait a minute, in that heat of the moment if you grab somebody, they can just turn around and start wailing on you. I told him to wait because we don't know what's going on yet," he says. Bobby was itching to intervene, though, because, as Roy says, "this guy was getting his ass whupped."

As if it weren't already serious, though, the incident was about to take a deadly turn. Roy noticed that one of the men doing the beating had a gun in his waistband. This is the exact type of situation that Roy and Bobby are supposed to break up. This is what they trained for, what they're out on the streets to resolve. Roy and Bobby both knew that they had to step in or someone was going to get killed.

Bobby made his presence known by shouting at the men doing the beating and telling them to break it up. They stopped but continued to yell obscenities at the victim while Roy tried to calm the situation down by talking to them. He wanted to keep their attention on him and away from the man they were assaulting. Bobby checked on the man, who was still awake but whose shirt was torn. He was woozy and bloody, with a bruised-up face. But this wasn't over; the three weren't done with their attack, no matter how much Roy tried to talk them down. Roy knew that he and Bobby would soon be viewed as in the way. Regardless, they persisted and pleaded with the men. Roy kept his eye on the gun. There was only one goal for Roy and Bobby at that moment: don't let this guy pull the gun out. The rest of the crowd didn't notice the gun, or if they did, they didn't react to it. A gun itself won't spark a panic, but pulling a trigger will.

Roy was able to get the armed man off to the side and kept his attention. Bobby focused on the other two. The man with the gun told Roy what happened. The guy they were beating hit his mother, and he "wasn't having that." Roy thought he was breaking through, but someone in the crowd said the police were coming. The armed man took off. Roy and Bobby were able to keep the other two there and discuss the issue more. Grateful that no one was killed in this situation, Roy and Bobby had to get more details to resolve the disagreement and make sure no retaliation followed.

Violence interruption is not a perfect science. Roy and his team are trained to think about safety first. They want to break up situations, but they have to be able to properly assess them before stepping in. This is hard to do in the midst of the conflict that they're witnessing. The goal is to de-escalate, ideally before a conflict becomes violent. They want to prevent any kind of violence, especially shootings. They have no power to arrest or prosecute, just their voices and influence. That's why they're also referred to as "credible messengers." Roy's voice carries weight. Since violence interrupters view violence as a disease that spreads, it's not just about the person who pulls the trigger and the victim who is shot or killed. The factors that contribute to the violence can't be ignored. Violence interrupters want to stop the spread.

How did the shooter get the weapon? Why were the shooter and the victim on the streets? What was the conflict about? Will there be retaliation? Who else was injured? There are a number of factors that violence interrupters have to grapple with. They use this information to try to prevent the next shooting. They know they can't stop every incident of violence. They don't have the ability to hold people accountable the way law enforcement can. Regardless of the flaws in the system, Roy is grateful for this work. He believes he's saved lives, and the organization he works for has become a place for the youth and adults to get out of the streets and do positive work in the community. He knows it's not the only answer to gun violence, but it's an important piece.

After the incident near the Louis Armstrong projects, over the next couple of years, Roy felt like the work had a significant positive impact on gun violence in the areas they worked in. He later became a manager in his organization, leading a group of violence interrupters. It's no surprise. Whether he's planning events, engaging with his colleagues, or guiding the young kids in the community, people listen. He's a natural leader. Even though it might not look like it, Roy admits that this work takes a toll. He has a schedule and is supposed to work on specific days during specific hours, but he views it as a 24/7 job. He'll be home spending time with his family but will constantly check his phone for messages or emails about things happening in the neighborhood.

Nationally, after a surge in 2015 and 2016, most major cities saw a decline in gun violence incidents during 2018 and 2019. Entering 2020, New York City was experiencing a decline in shootings and homicides, which coincided with what was happening in other cities across the country. From 2017 to 2019, New York City saw some of its lowest crime and incarceration rates ever. Roy remembers the early months of 2020 being celebratory for him and his team. They had gone from October 2019 to January 2020 without a single shooting in their catchment area (the radius where he

does intervention work). This wasn't just isolated to their immediate location; other sites that used violence interrupters were seeing similar extended periods of peace.

Though it's always a concern, the numbers suggested that
shootings were declining nationally. One of the last events Roy remembers from early 2020 is when he and his team put together a
community gathering after a young girl was jumped by a few teenage boys. Though the group primarily deals with community
gun violence, this incident caught the attention of folks in the
neighborhood. "The community was in an uproar about it. Many
were calling on [us] and asking us what we were going to do about
it. We decided it made sense for us to do a community healing
response," he says. They descended on the corner in Brooklyn
where the attack took place. A large group of residents was at the
scene as folks took turns speaking to the community, around 100
people, including kids, adults and the elderly.

Using a megaphone, the violence-prevention workers and residents spoke pointedly to the crowd. Condemning the attack, they
called it unacceptable, making eye contact with any young men
they saw in the audience. "Your parents did not raise you to be-
have like this," one woman said, which led to some applause. They
also stressed the need for more community harmony and accountability among adults when dealing with kids. The gathering was
down the block from a police station and drew the attention of
some officers, who initially tried to break it up before they realized what was happening. While the speakers didn't pull any
punches, the atmosphere was peaceful and heartwarming. This
moment has stuck in Roy's head because of what it represented
at the time. It was just a community that cared about its residents,
responding to something terrible that had happened. No one was
making excuses, but there was a feeling of compassion in the
crowd. Roy did not know that this would be the last time his team
would gather in a large crowd for a couple of years—a few weeks

later, an unprecedented citywide lockdown would commence in response to a new respiratory virus.

The first confirmed coronavirus case in New York City was on March 1, 2020, after a woman returned to her Manhattan home from Iran on February 25. By this point, fear of the virus was rapidly growing throughout the country and the rest of the world. Italy's lockdown in February served as a warning sign for many Americans. If anyone was paying close attention, though, there were plenty of other warning signs for what was to come. Healthcare professionals were aware of the virus in late 2019. The World Health Organization began making announcements concerning the virus in January 2020. The second confirmed New York case came from a New Rochelle lawyer on March 3. The next day, nine other people who had interacted with the lawyer tested positive. New Rochelle quickly became one of the early epicenters of the virus in the United States.

In early March people were scrambling. Many were stocking up on groceries, toilet paper, and hand sanitizer. Others—the ones who had the means to do so—were leaving major cities and returning to their family homes. Everyone else had to stay where they were. Folks were trying to prepare as much as they could for the virus. On March 11, the World Health Organization declared a global pandemic. Soon after, President Donald Trump declared COVID-19 a national pandemic. On March 15, a stay-at-home order began, and the country was locked down for months.

It's difficult to fully explain what the early months of the pandemic were like for US citizens. The foot traffic that large cities usually saw was gone. Curfews were put in place. Many suburban and rural areas resembled ghost towns. Major corporations sent their workers home. Small businesses were temporarily closed. Some of them would permanently shutter. Students had to attend school remotely. The court system was closed. Jails released inmates. Many social service agencies transitioned their employees to working from home.

Hospitals quickly became overwhelmed with people infected by the virus. There wasn't enough staff or equipment to properly care for those who became ill. But it wasn't just hospitals: resources for all city- and state-run agencies became scarce. The pandemic also halted the country's economy. People lost their jobs, their homes, and their savings. The death tolls were staggering. By the end of March 2020, there were over 4,000 people dead in the United States from COVID. By the end of September, it was nearly 200,000. By March 2021, the number had climbed to over 500,000. It felt like the pandemic might never end. Nationally, there was a sense of existential dread. If you had some money or some level of privilege then the effects weren't as bad, but if you were poor it was detrimental. No matter where someone was or who they were, they felt it in some way.

Roy and his team certainly did. They were no longer out in the streets as much. Their face-to-face meetings were limited. All big group gatherings were canceled. They now had to do the majority of their community work through texting and phone calls, which made it more difficult. One thing his organization did was provide community members with personal protective equipment (PPE)—masks, hand sanitizer, gloves, and other supplies—which was hard to come by at the time. Roy says their focus was as much on COVID as it was on gun violence.

It became clear which communities were going to be the most affected by COVID: poor minority neighborhoods across the country, the very kind of community that Roy works in. "It really exposed the conditions of our communities," Roy says. "The people that were already struggling just started to struggle more." The public health crisis revealed just how vast inequality was in the country, from health care to housing to education.

In the initial weeks following the stay-at-home orders, some major cities saw drops in crime. During the last two weeks of March 2020, New York City saw a 20 percent decrease in overall crime. Los Angeles experienced an 11 percent decrease in crime for the entire month of March 2020. The early crime numbers might have felt like a silver lining in these neighborhoods, but people couldn't predict what would happen next.

Just like New York City, Chicago locked down on March 21. LaTanya Gordon is a lifelong Chicago resident. She raised six children on the South Side. When COVID hit, LaTanya was a frontline worker who was employed as a caretaker for the elderly. She couldn't work from home. The South Side of Chicago is notorious for its struggle with gun violence, both past and present. The Gordon family was not naive about that, which is why LaTanya made it a habit to listen to the police scanner while driving.

She raised her kids to defend themselves, and her fourth-oldest son, Tyler Malden, was no exception. If you tried him, he was ready to fight. LaTanya was close with all her children, including Tyler, who was 20. He had two jobs, working at FedEx and a neighborhood bowling alley. Though he had some run-ins with the law, he mostly kept to himself. "He wasn't a troublemaker, but he wasn't a perfect kid either," LaTanya says. He was like a lot of other young men, drawn to clothes, girls, cars, and music.

On April 6, 2020, LaTanya was returning home from a long shift. She had her scanner on and heard that there was a shooting in South Deering, the neighborhood she lived in. She listened to the details but quickly moved on. Just another shooting in the constant cycle of violence. She, like many others, was used to hearing news like that.

When she got home, however, the police called her. This shooting wasn't just another random occurrence in the neighborhood. Her son Tyler was the victim. Before she'd even gotten the call, he was dead at the hospital. LaTanya knew plenty of young Black men who were killed in her community, but she had never dealt with it directly. From a big-picture perspective, Tyler's death was inconsequential. LaTanya was just another mother who lost a child to inner-city gun violence. A week before the stay-at-home orders went into effect in Chicago, there were 25 shooting incidents. In the first week of the stay-at-home orders, it rose to 41. The next week there were 40, including Tyler's. LaTanya doesn't know exactly what happened, but she believes her son was targeted.

Tyler's brother Terrance was 15 at the time. Like his older brother, he didn't back down from anyone. Whatever happened on the streets between Tyler and his assailant, Terrance knew about it. In the months after the shooting, Terrance was open in public about his feelings toward the shooter. He would talk badly about him in the streets. LaTanya cautioned him to keep his thoughts private and not bring too much attention to himself. She wanted him to let the police do their job and arrest the shooter. She worried about his safety. Terrance was hurting, though. Tyler was his older brother. He looked up to him. He wrestled with him, played video games with him, and sought his approval. They were close, as close as two brothers could be. Terrance knew his brother wasn't in a gang, but he was around enough gang members for rivals to get the wrong idea. After all, so was Terrance. In their neighborhood, it's hard to avoid gang members if you're going to be outside. Just being friends with the wrong person can put a target on your back.

Terrance wasn't a punk. At 15 years old, he had gall. He didn't just badmouth the shooter, he went after him verbally. He openly called him a coward. As far as Terrance saw it, there was no reason for his brother to have been killed. He wasn't thinking about what the consequences could be if he spoke out. He didn't care. He just wanted people on the streets to know that he wasn't afraid of this guy. Months went by, and gun violence was spiking in the city. In July 2020, Tyler's murder was still unsolved and the family was frustrated, including Terrance, who remained vocal about his thoughts on the murder.

On July 10, at around a quarter of five in the afternoon, Terrance was walking down South Hoxie Avenue in the Jeffrey Manor neighborhood of Chicago when a white Audi drove up next to him. His street instincts would have told him something was up. As Terrance looked in the direction of the car, someone opened one of the doors and shot at him five times. He tried to run away but was hit in the back by one of the bullets. The car sped off. In agony, the kid crawled into an alley. In the direst situation of his life, he called his mother, gasping for air while he told her what had happened. LaTanya panicked and called 911. She told the authorities where Terrance was. It took them a few minutes to arrive, during which LaTanya stayed on the phone with her son, telling him to hang on and that help was on the way. It was too late though. Terrance died shortly after he was taken to the hospital.

In just four months, LaTanya lost two sons to gun violence.

After everything she did to keep her family safe, the scanner was probably just the tip of the iceberg. "I'm sick of it. I'm tired of it. We talk about Black Lives Matter, but I'm sick and tired of what's going on in these streets," Erikka Gordon, the victims' aunt, said at the time. In 2019 there were 495 homicides in Chicago. That number exploded to 769 in 2020, which included Tyler's and Terrance's murders. Most of those murders were done with a gun. Chicago is usually pointed to as an exception for gun violence. The numbers in the city tend to be so bad compared with other places that it can be easy to ignore if you don't live in the city. The year LaTanya lost two of her sons was different. Almost every city felt the weight of pervasive gun violence.

If there was a thought that the increased gun violence seen in Atlanta in 2020 was going to be some sort of outlier, that was quickly dismissed in 2021. Just ask Davante Griffin. Davante is built solid; he played football in high school. Even-keeled and amiable, there's a steadiness to his presence. His son Deuce is his everything. When he looks at Deuce and tells him to "say cheese" for a photo, the kid lets out the biggest and most adorable bubbly smile. He's a carefree and happy toddler. There's a gleam in Davante's eyes when he hugs and kisses his son, and it's clear he's incredibly proud to be a father.

Growing up, Davante lived in a few different areas in and around Atlanta. By his count, it was more than five different neighborhoods, mainly on the east side of the city, where the streets are "hot." He has stories for days, about his friends, his family, and his own experiences. He'll write a book one day to lay it all out. His father wasn't around, and his mother died of cancer when he was 20. His stepfather was killed by police when he was a kid. His family was close-knit, but a lot of that changed after his mother died. "She was the only person that was always there for me and my siblings. Family members were around for a while after she died, but that didn't last long," he says with indifference.

Davante certainly doesn't view himself as a gangster. "You gotta have the mindset to overcome the streets and look past them," he says. He's never sold drugs, never been in a gang, and never robbed anyone. But he knows the streets. He grew up in them, and he has seen everything. He's seen people get shot. He has relatives doing life sentences for murder and for selling drugs. Seeing all of this taught him a lot. "You gotta watch what you're doing. It teaches you how to move out here," Davante says.

The one experience he never had was getting shot. "I've come close; I've been shot at before, but I had never been hit." That all changed in March 2021. Davante was at home with a handful of friends and his brother in Henry County, about 45 minutes south of Atlanta. "That's the outskirts, nothing goes down out there," he says. After he spent the day with his son, Deuce's mother, Dejia, came to pick him up. Davante spoke with her outside. They weren't dating anymore and Davante wanted to discuss getting back together. Dejia told him she wasn't ready. She needed to figure things out. "I wasn't buying that shit though," Davante says. After she left with Deuce, he was pissed off. He went back inside and vented to his brother and a couple of friends. "If we gonna be together, we might as well figure it out," he told them. Instead of just sitting in his anger, he decided to take the stress out on video games. He went upstairs to his room, closed the door, turned on his 75-inch TV, put his headphones on, and got to work on *Call of Duty*. "I just zoned out in front of the TV," he says. Then he heard a loud noise.

He thought it must've been coming from the TV. *Call of Duty* isn't a quiet game, especially when you have the headphones blasting, because it contains a lot of shooting, shouting, and explosions. Davante heard the noise again and realized it was not from the game. The noises got louder, and he understood that they were coming from downstairs. *Doom doom doom doom doom doom.* Like someone was banging on a door or a table. He turned the game down to be 100 percent clear that the sounds were not coming from the TV.

They weren't.

At first, he thought there was an argument or a fight happening between his friends. They fight all the time. Sometimes it's jokes; sometimes it's serious. Davante figured this must be one of the serious ones. He thought, "Let me go downstairs and see what was up." As he got up, though, the noises grew louder, like loud footsteps coming up the stairs. He swung his door open to one of his friends rushing up the stairs, out of breath. "Someone breaking into ya'll crib," he yelled. "Yeah okay," Davante said sarcastically. But it wasn't until he saw someone else come up the stairs—in a mask with a gun—that the reality set in. "Oh, this shit real."

Davante quickly closed his door and looked for his gun. He likes to keep it out of his son's reach, and he forgot where he put it during Deuce's visit. Just as he heard the robber say to his friend, "Tell your man to come out of the room," Davante found the gun on top of his dresser. Davante is naturally stoic, but in that moment he looked frantic. He held the gun up, the barrel parallel with his nose, and he stood by the light and the door. He tried to control his shaky breaths. Thinking on his feet, Davante turned the light off in his room. "Tell your man to come out the room," the would-be robber repeated. Davante thought to himself, "Don't worry, nigga, I'm coming." He slowly pushed the door open, pointed his gun out, and fired.

But in an instant, he was shot, almost at the same moment he pulled the trigger. He was hit in the leg. The pain was instant, though he believes his adrenaline kept it from being worse. Davante jumped back and crawled into the closet. He looked around, unsure of what to do next. Then, when he saw a T-shirt on the ground, it came to him. He tied it around his leg to stop the bleeding. He had the gun pointed at the door still, ready to fire more. Loud screams came from the hallway. He thought it might have been the robber screaming from being shot, but it was actually his friend, who was shot five times.

With all the noise, the robbers left the house, before Davante could get out of the closet. They took nothing with them. The police came not too long after. Davante and his friend were taken in separate ambulances to the hospital. On the ride there, Davante was just trying to stay awake. "I had heard that you could die from a gunshot wound to the leg, so I didn't want to close my eyes," he says. As he tried to stay awake in the back of the ambulance, his mind was racing. "What if I don't see my son again? Is my boy going to make it? Am I getting arrested for this? What if those guys try to find me again? If this is it, I need to hear my son's voice one more time."

Once he got to the hospital, he called Dejia. She was still mad about their discussion, so she wasn't answering. He had to call his sister and ask her to call Dejia. When Dejia found out Davante had been shot, she panicked. She lost her father when she was 2, the same age Deuce was at the time. She was petrified. She couldn't imagine her son growing up without his dad. She tried to call him back, but the hospital had given Davante drugs for the pain by this point. She called all the hospitals but none of them would give her information. It turns out the police listed him under a different name when he was admitted, to protect him. Dejia got in her car and drove around to different hospitals, but she couldn't find him. It was a hopeless and helpless feeling. After trying several hospitals, she just sat in her car on the side of the highway and waited for his call. He had to be alive; he simply had to be.

Hours later, he finally called her back. Miraculously, no one was killed. Davante still doesn't know who the culprits were. It was a good thing he had his gun, but he wonders if his friend still would have gotten shot if he didn't fire first. He doesn't regret it, though. "You shoot at me, I'm shooting back," he says. This was one of the 750 shooting incidents citywide in 2021, which was a 6 percent increase from 2020. In 2020, 157 people were killed in Atlanta, most by gun violence. In 2021 the number was 158.

In 2022, a new hot-button topic was grabbing people's attention, and journalists, pundits, academics, experts, and criminologists were all circling it: the uptick in shooting numbers was becoming too unrelenting to ignore. This was an election year, and public safety was surely going to be a sticking point for the upcoming midterms. But that wasn't the only driver of the increased focus, as several gun violence tragedies in 2022 also grabbed the nation's attention. In a mass shooting in Buffalo, New York, a white supremacist gunman traveled over three hours to a supermarket in a majority-Black neighborhood, where he shot 10 people to death. The country barely had time to process it before a worse tragedy happened in the South. An elementary school in Uvalde, Texas, became the site of the third-deadliest school shooting in American history when a gunman killed 19 students and 2 teachers.

With these massacres happening less than two weeks apart, the country zeroed in on gun violence, particularly mass shootings. Incidents in which multiple people are killed, especially innocent souls like schoolchildren and shoppers, will draw everyone's attention, regardless of where someone stands on gun control and gun policy. With the nation focused on large-scale tragedies like those in Buffalo and Uvalde, the daily mass shootings in the hood are often ignored.

In 2022, Roy felt the weight of what was happening in New York City. The app he uses to track crime in his neighborhood was constantly alerting him of new incidents. Many people felt like New York was heading back to the old days when gun crimes happened almost everywhere in the city. That didn't—and would never—stop New Yorkers from being out and about in the summertime.

Darius Lee and his family took advantage of that time. He was a rising senior at Houston Baptist University (HBU) in Texas, where he was a member of the basketball team and studied kinesiology. The six-foot-six, 230-pound guard was a standout at HBU, averaging 18 points and 8 rebounds a game during his second year in the program. He set a school record with 52 points against McNeese State during his junior season. Though he was a guard, Lee could bump down low with strong post-ups, hook shots, and up-and-under moves. On the perimeter, he had a nice little herky-jerky game, and because of his size, he was difficult to stop when he got a head of steam to the basket. If you fouled him, he could live at the free-throw line. During the summer of 2022, Darius was back in Harlem, New York—his hometown—with his family. As a local legend, he spent some time speaking to the players at St. Raymond High School for Boys in the Bronx, where he had attended school.

Residents were enjoying the holiday weekend; it was June-teenth and Father's Day. Many celebrated at cookouts, which are a sight to behold in New York over the summer. Kids run around playing. Parents and adults talk or argue while they hold a plate of food. Intense card games are easy to find at these gatherings. If not cards, then it's dominos. The cookout could be scheduled to start at two o'clock but people won't start showing up till four. Someone has to man the grill and take orders. Burgers, hot dogs, wings, chicken, and salads accompanied by sodas, juices, and of course alcohol. If you're smart, you'll pack and store your to-go plate before you actually eat at the cookout. The cookouts are held on the sidewalks, in the parks, or in people's backyards. Darius was at one near East 139th Street and 5th Avenue in Harlem, right next to the East River.

The cookout started in the afternoon but, typical of these events, it went on through the evening, into the night, and then into the dead of night. Around twelve thirty in the morning, the atmosphere changed a little bit. There weren't as many kids around, and the cooking was still going on but not to the same degree as earlier in the day. It can still be an enjoyable time, but there's more room for conflict.

No one is sure exactly what happened; there were a lot of people there, including a handful of gang members, but the celebration still overshadowed any issues that went on. That is, until a fight broke out between a group of men and there were gunshots.

Not a few or even a few dozen of them—150 shots were fired.

People dispersed quickly. Many of them ran away on a nearby highway ramp. Some of them were hit by gunfire. Nine people were shot, including Darius, who died later at the hospital. He was 21. Everyone else survived. Authorities later confirmed that the shooting was the result of a conflict between "two heavily armed groups." Darius was not an intended target.

"I had a little boy come up to me yesterday and tapped my shoulder, he was standing over the picture [of Darius] we have up in front of the building," Taren Weaver, Darius's mother, said after her son was killed. "And he pointed to the picture and he was like 'do you miss him? Because I miss him.' It broke my heart to hear him say that." No one was arrested for Darius's death. The mass shooting in Harlem didn't have as many fatalities as the ones in Buffalo and Uvalde, but it was another incident in which gunfire erupted among an unsuspecting group of people. There were 646 mass shootings in 2022.

Contextualizing the gun violence numbers since 2020 can be difficult. There are so many ways to break it all down: total deaths, number of shooting incidents, types of incidents, age group, the racial breakdown of victims and known perpetrators, where the shootings happen, when the shootings happen, the rate of shooting homicides per 100,000 people, and so on. Some data points are less reliable and less useful than others. There isn't a national government database that tracks shooting incidents and deaths in real time. Only nonprofit groups and think tanks do that. The government record of these deaths (which is compiled by the FBI) comes out a year after the fact.

The total numbers are a good place to start. Some of the numbers vary depending on the source, but for the most part the organizations that track these numbers are reliable. Before 2020, America was already the leader in gun violence deaths in the world. It has the highest murder rate per 100,000 out of all the high-income nations. An average of 40,000 Americans die from gun violence each year, which is around 110 per day.

In 2018, 39,740 people were killed by gun violence. This includes homicides, suicides, unintentional shootings, and legal intervention or law enforcement shootings, according to the data from the Centers for Disease Control and Prevention (CDC), which is one of the more reliable sources for this information. The CDC reports 39,707 firearm deaths in 2019. The number went up to 43,675 in 2020. It increased in 2021 to 47,286, which was the highest total number of gun deaths in the country in over 30 years.

The Gun Violence Archive is a nonprofit organization that tracks gun violence incidents. It's the only place to get real-time national gun violence data. They have a dedicated staff that uses daily law enforcement numbers and media reports to compile their data. "We utilize automated queries, manual research through over 7,500 sources from local and state police, media, data aggregates, government and other sources daily. Each incident is verified by both initial researchers and secondary validation processes," their website says. They report a total of 45,118 gun violence deaths in 2021 as of August 2023. For context, their 2020 number is 43,747 at the same point in August 2023. There were over 44,000 firearm deaths in 2022, with over 20,200 of them being firearm homicides. The organization updates these numbers as they get more information.

Percentage-wise, gun homicides went up 39 percent in 2020 compared with 2019. They went up 25 percent compared with 2015 and 43 percent compared with 2010. Overall, the homicide rate in 2020 was 30 percent higher nationally than it was in 2019, according to a report from the Council on Criminal Justice (CCJ), a nonprofit criminal justice think tank that "advance[s] understanding of the criminal justice policy challenges facing the nation and build[s] consensus for solutions based on facts, evidence, and fundamental principles of justice." The FBI's numbers are identical. Their report on crime in 2020 showed that homicides went up by 30% in 2020 compared with 2019. The murder rate increase from 2019 to 2020 was the largest single-year increase since the 1960s. Cities like Milwaukee, Portland, Minneapolis, Chicago, Fort Worth, and Omaha had some of the highest murder rate increases from 2019 to 2020.

Total homicide numbers across the country don't exclusively include gun deaths. When police departments report their homicide numbers, they include all types of killing. But the majority of homicides committed in the United States are done with a gun. In 2020, 79 percent of all US murders involved a firearm.

While the data may vary from place to place, what's clear is that the problem got worse in 2020, shortly after the pandemic began. Some data do suggest that gun violence was already off to a bad start at the beginning of 2020. It continued to rise in 2021 before dipping in 2022 and into 2023, though the numbers were still higher than in 2019. When we see the national numbers, it's easy to assume that gun violence just increased all over and that neighborhoods where it doesn't usually happen became cesspools for violence. What actually happened, especially in the first year of the pandemic, was that gun violence worsened in the areas where it was already a problem.

"According to every bit of evidence, the rises were occurring in the very same communities where homicide rates have traditionally been exceptionally high," Rick Rosenfeld, a renowned criminologist, says. Professor Rosenfeld is a part of CCJ and was a coauthor of many of their crime trend reports released since 2020. He adds that the nature of the homicides didn't change much either. "What happened was the level of homicides in these neighborhoods that have traditionally been elevated, that went up."

Historically, poor Black communities have been plagued by gun violence. It's so much a part of this country that people barely bat an eye at it. It's expected and accepted at this point. David M. Kennedy, in his 2011 book *Don't Shoot: One Man, a Street Fellowship, and the End of Violence in Inner-City America*, brilliantly explains the dynamic: "[Black Americans] are not being killed by the cops. They are being killed by each other. Black Americans are about a seventh of America. They do about half America's killing and half America's violent dying—young men most of both."

That quote still sums it up. Black Americans are much more likely to fall victim to gun violence than any other racial group in this country. They're 10 times more likely to die as a result of gun homicides and 18 times more likely to be the victim of gun assault injuries than any other race. The leading cause of death for Black males in America ages 1 to 44 is homicide. Despite only being 13 percent of the population, Black Americans make up a third of all gun violence deaths. For Black women, gun violence is the second leading cause of death. Firearm homicides went up 39 percent from 2019 to 2020 among Black people, which was the highest increase for any racial group between the two years. There are more Black homicide victims in the country than any other group. Nationally, the leading cause of death for white men is heart disease. Many racial disparities exist in America, but none is more striking than the disparity in who gets shot.

Intraracial violence (violence committed within the same race) occurs for all races. White people overwhelmingly kill other white people, but the rates at which Black people kill each other and die are disproportionate. For example, in Maryland, Black men make up 15 percent of the population but account for 82 percent of the gun violence victims. In Washington, DC, 96 percent of all shooting and homicide victims are Black. The city is 46 percent Black. Think about that: almost all the people who die from guns in the nation's capital are Black people. If you look at New York City, the data show that since 2008, 95 percent of shooting victims have been either Black or Hispanic.

This problem reaches everyone, but it places a much larger strain on the Black community.

There are many misconceptions about what drives gun violence in the country. A lot of the violence is the result of gang conflicts and fights between rival drug crews, but it's also driven by confrontations between other people that get out of hand. For instance, a couple of guys could be hanging out on the block. One of them makes a disrespectful comment toward the other that gets the "ohhhhh" reaction from everyone else. Instead of the insulted person saying something clever back or using their fists, they pull out a gun and shoot.

Another misunderstanding is that it's a bunch of young people running around and shooting. The reality is most shooters and victims are between the ages of 20 and 29. Sure, there are some kids pulling triggers, but it's mostly grown men.

Gun violence rose in pretty much every major city in the country in 2020, but it didn't rise across the entire city. It rose in the dense, disenfranchised neighborhoods in the inner city, where Black people live. "The lives that are most directly threatened by this are lives that we don't value as much as other lives; they're the most distant, disenfranchised, and disadvantaged people in society," Thomas Abt, a crime researcher and author of *Bleeding Out: The Devastating Consequences of Urban Violence—and a Bold New Plan for Peace in the Streets*, says. All of those problems existed before 2020. When gun violence intensified, no other population group carried the toll the way Black and brown communities had to.

"The worst effects were felt in the communities with traditionally high rates of gun violence, and these are traditionally communities of concentrated disadvantages," Daniel Webster, of the Johns Hopkins Center for Gun Violence Prevention and Policy in the Bloomberg School of Public Health, says. "They're primarily African American communities that for a very long time had disinvestment and a variety of structural challenges." When the numbers started to rise in 2020, Professor Webster was one of the main researchers whom reporters went to for perspective. He's one of the premier experts in the gun-violence prevention field.

Contrary to popular belief, mass shootings happen within these neighborhoods all the time. The FBI doesn't directly define what is considered a mass shooting, but the most accepted definition is an incident in which four or more people are shot or killed, not including the shooter. In 2020 there were 610 mass shootings in the United States, and in 2021 there were 691. The mass shootings that get everyone's attention can be defined as high-fatality mass shootings. Yet mass shootings only account for around 1 percent of all firearm deaths in the country. Shootings in the hood drive the carnage.

While the number of police shootings pales in comparison, it is around 1,000 people per year and has stayed consistent since 2020. These include lawful and unlawful incidents. It's important to note that the data on police shootings are flawed and difficult to track because of a lack of transparency across all US law enforcement agencies. The most reliable data only go back to 2013.

The CDC reported that firearms became the leading cause of death for children and teenagers in 2020, bypassing the previous leader, which was car accidents. Black kids were already overexposed to gun violence compared with white kids. In 2020, the gap widened. Suicides make up a large percentage of gun-related deaths, along with community gun violence. In 2019 there were 23,941 firearm suicides. Surprisingly, the number has remained steady, with 24,292 in 2020 and 26,328 in 2021.

Domestic violence coupled with access to a firearm is always a concern, and 2020 was no exception. Over half of all intimate partner murders are done with a gun. The CCJ reported an 8 percent increase in domestic violence incidents following the stay-at-home orders that came in 2020. There was an increase in calls to domestic violence helplines. These facts suggest a very dangerous situation.

In terms of other types of crime, aggravated assaults and gun assaults also went up in 2020 and 2021. Motor vehicle thefts would see a big spike in 2020 and 2021, but by the end of 2021 they started to trend downward. Larceny, burglaries, and drug offenses all went down in 2020 and 2021. People often make a mistake when discussing crime and gun violence because they fail to see a distinction between the two, or rather between crime and violent crime. Gun violence is a crime, but it's not in the same category as something like property damage, which occurs with much more frequency than gun violence. There needs to be some distinction between overall crime and violent crime like gun violence, especially considering that the data on other types of crime aren't great. Homicide data are fairly reliable.

It's generally understood in the expert community that rates per 100,000 are a more reliable data point for tracking trends over time than using total numbers. That being said, it's one of the more misunderstood metrics used when examining gun deaths. The national firearm homicide rate per 100,000 was 4.3 in 2019. In 2020 it was 6.4, and in 2021 it was 6.8. States like Mississippi, Louisiana, Wyoming, and Alabama have the highest rates of murder. But Mississippi had 576 homicides in 2020, whereas Chicago had over 769. Chicago is 234 square miles, while Mississippi is 48,000 square miles. So while the rate per 100,000 may be higher in a state like Mississippi, more people are dying in some cities than in entire states.

The rate per 100,000 is a critical data point, it just gets framed in a way that's not useful. It's used as a way to dismiss the surge in murders that happened in 2020. "As we got more data and did a really careful look, gun homicides increased almost everywhere in the country," Professor Webster says.

The increase in rural areas was around 28 percent. It's still the disenfranchised parts of those rural areas that were hit the hardest, however. "It's always more concentrated in poor communities, which are communities of color. Pretty much any issue hits those communities the hardest," Paul Carrillo, the Community Violence Initiative director at the Giffords Law Center to Prevent Gun Violence, says.

The rate per 100,000 is useful for zooming in on a specific area or neighborhood, especially the smaller ones. New York City, which has a population of around 8 million people, had 319 murders in 2019 and 462 in 2020, a 45 percent increase. The number went up to 485 in 2021. In 2019, 776 shooting incidents happened across the city. That number drastically went up to 1,531 in 2020 and rose again in 2021 to 1,562. The homicide rate in the city is around 6 per 100,000 residents.

Youngstown, Ohio, a small city about an hour northwest of Pittsburgh, has a population of around 64,000. It is similar to other small midwestern cities. In 2019, the city had 13 murders. That went up to 28 in 2020 and went up again to 30 in 2021. Shooting incidents rose across those three years as well, going from 58 to 98 and then up to 138 in 2021. On the surface, those low numbers can be dismissed, but in a small city, each one of those deaths is felt hard. "None of us are immune to it. There are only so many schools, so many barbershops, so many grocery stores, so many jobs," Youngstown mayor Jamael Tito Brown says. "The closer you look you can always find somebody who knows somebody connected to you." Their homicide rate is around 46 per 100,000 residents. Such numbers are a good reminder that as much as this is a national problem, gun violence is truly a local issue—a hyperlocal issue at that. This means it needs to be dealt with individually in each city. Sometimes half of the violent crime in a city is happening in a three-block radius in a poor neighborhood.

These numbers represent a lot. They represent all the family members and loved ones who have to bury a relative or friend. They represent the emotional weight that survivors have to carry for the rest of their lives. They represent the burden that's placed on law enforcement to hold the killers accountable and make sure they see justice. They represent the burden that's placed on everyday hardworking citizens who have to live in these communities. They represent the toll that's placed on social services and community groups. They represent the financial cost that follows.

America is all about money. What people don't realize is that gun violence costs money. It costs the country billions of dollars every year, though estimates vary from $280 billion to $550 billion a year. "Gun violence, particularly murderous gun violence, is just extraordinarily costly, upwards of 10 million per homicide. The way it directly impacts property values, tax revenues, insurance costs and all of these different things cannot be ignored," Thomas says. "What we see is when it gets bad enough, it can literally strangle the economic livelihood of a city. It's a direct threat to a city's prosperity."

In his book, Thomas Abt superbly breaks down what that $10 million cost is. He describes both direct and indirect costs. Direct costs include those incurred in the hospital system, court system, and incarceration system, as well as property damage. The indirect costs are trickier to quantify, but they tend to be greater than the direct costs. For example, the value of buildings and homes usually plummets in neighborhoods where violence surges. This leads to fewer people going to the area, and that's where the real financial cost of gun violence manifests itself. Think about the people who live on blocks where shootings happen on a regular basis. Daily gunshots destroy any chance of building wealth or sustainability. For Black people, it inhibits the chance of prosperity in their communities.

There are those who look at the numbers and compare them to what was happening in the 1990s when crime and gun violence were skyrocketing. The number of murders in New York City since 2020 doesn't come close to those in the 1990s, which were in the thousands. Some cities, like Philadelphia, St. Louis, Minneapolis, and Memphis, did eclipse their numbers from the 1990s, but nationally the issue is not as bad as it was during that period. Most of the United States is safe, and most major US cities are safe. Still, the rise from 2019 to 2020 was unprecedented and cannot be ignored. In the years since gun violence became more lethal, victims have died at the scene a lot more than they did decades ago. Beyond that, the problem is still directly affecting the most vulnerable communities, as it was over 20 years ago. It would be hard to tell LaTanya that gun violence isn't as bad today as it was in the 1990s.

With all this being said, the big question is why? Why did the circumstances around the COVID pandemic make this issue worse? Regardless of what pundits and journalists want to say today, there's never been one answer to what drives this issue.

People point to poverty, police, a lack of family structure, and a lack of accountability and self-responsibility. Everyone wants to find the one reason so they can develop the one solution. But since there isn't one reason, none of the singular solutions work on their own. "When you look at everything, the surge that we saw was predictable. It's not unfathomable that we had this surge in gun violence, especially given where it happened," Dr. Shani Buggs, a public health professor and prominent gun violence researcher, says.

Everything was upended around the country in 2020. There wasn't a corner of the population that did not feel it. What happened in the disenfranchised minority communities, though, could be described as a perfect storm.

2

The Perfect Storm

Unlike many others born and raised in Bed-Stuy during the 1980s, Roy came from a stable home. He lived in a three-family brownstone. Today brownstone homes in Brooklyn can go for a few million dollars, but back then they were much more affordable. Before Roy was born, his family moved up to New York City from the South. He was raised by his mother, grandmother, and great-grandmother. They all lived in the house together, along with a handful of cousins.

"There weren't any men in the house," Roy recalls. "My grandfather had already passed away. So my mom and grandmothers were the matriarchs and the patriarchs." Roy had to take on the man's responsibilities. From an early age, he went to the store for everyone. He would get groceries, get the Sunday paper, and run all types of errands. He didn't just do this for the people in his home; he did it for old folks on the block as well. It was common for him to carry four copies of the Sunday paper and distribute them on the block.

"Basically, I grew up around a lot of elderly people," he says. "I grew up in a very loving environment. I grew up with that concept of caring and concern." His street was a real community. There was a block association and they always had parties. It was very festive. There was certainly crime, violence, and drug use happening in his neighborhood, but it didn't outweigh the communal aspect that his particular block had. As Roy puts it, this was before the crack epidemic "became big." His mother was 17 when she had him. She was still out trying to finish school and find a job when he was young, so his grandmothers were the ones who guided him.

Though his grandparents were a positive example for Roy, as they got older, they couldn't keep up with him and his cousins. With the younger parents not around, things took a turn. One day, when Roy was about 9, he and his cousins were playing on the top floor of their brownstone. They lit some matches they had found and accidentally started a fire. No one was killed, but the fire essentially destroyed the house. They tried to stay there afterward, but there was no electricity and no heat, and they had little access to hot water. "We just couldn't really stay in there after that so that's when we moved out," he says. At first, he and his mother lived with one of his aunts, but then they went to a shelter outside Bed-Stuy, in Brownsville. It was at the shelter that Roy saw the real despair in his community.

When he lived in the shelter, getting to school in Bed-Stuy was more difficult. Soon, he started to miss school. After the shelter, Roy and his mom moved to a small apartment in Bed-Stuy, where he saw even more violence and drug use. Then they moved again, this time to a housing project. "We moved from a community-type atmosphere to a shelter and now to the projects. It's now a different ballgame," he says. "A whole different ballgame. That fire changed everything."

On a daily basis, Roy saw people pee in the elevator, which wasn't as bad as seeing the addicts smoke crack in the hallways and stairwells. He had to step on crack vials when he walked through his building. It was a far cry from what he knew. He started cutting school and hanging out on the block. It became difficult to ignore the streets. In a way, this new world was enticing to him. He saw guys out in the neighborhood shooting dice, doing pull-ups on the street signs, and playing the knockout game (a game typically played by kids and teens in which they run up to someone and sucker punch them in an attempt to knock them out). On Fridays, the older guys would hang out, drink, and smoke. They had all the girls around them. Roy never saw things like this in the little community he had on the old block. This new environment was cool. He wanted to be a part of it. He didn't want to be the square who didn't leave his apartment.

Roy went to classes until high school. That's when he couldn't ignore the call of the streets anymore. "I'll never forget the first time it really happened," he says. One night, when he was around 14, he rode bikes with a friend of his. Afterward, Roy was headed home when the friend, who was about to go somewhere else, asked him if he wanted to hold his gun overnight. It was a .25 ACP handgun. Excited, Roy said yes. He brought the gun to his apartment and sat in his room with it. He wanted to test it out but noticed that there were only two bullets in the clip. He was afraid that his friend would be upset if he shot one of the last two bullets. But his curiosity got the best of him. Around two o'clock that morning, he went outside his building and shot the gun up in the air. "It was really over from there," he says.

From then on he went from carrying guns, to shooting at people, to robbing people and getting in shoot-outs. "I was full-fledged in the streets now," he says. There was a lot his mother didn't know, but on the block, everyone knew him. He was a stickup kid. He had a real rep. If you were in the streets, you knew not to mess with him and his boys. It all caught up with him, though. At age 16 he was arrested for multiple armed robberies. The judge gave him 23 years. As if going to prison weren't enough, his mother died a month after he was sentenced. Two months after that his grandmother died. "It all just came crashing down on me," he says. Roy doesn't blame anyone but himself for the things he did as a youth that led him to prison. He wishes he just made better decisions. But he also acknowledges how the circumstances around him led to some of the choices he made. A poor neighborhood in one city may look different structurally and aesthetically from the one in Bed-Stuy, but they all struggle with the same problems.

Resources are hard to come by. There's a lack of jobs in these communities. Community centers, reliable health care, reliable housing, and reliable social services like mental health services are sparse. There is a lack of youth programs and after-school programs, and the schools themselves are already poorly funded. There's more stress in poor communities and more financial pressure. The police are not equipped to handle the structural issues. Their job is to police the neighborhoods and enforce the law, not serve as social workers. They already have a tense relationship with the residents in these communities. Of course, there are some community-led efforts to address all the inequalities, but many of them are underfunded and undersupported. And who primarily lives in these areas across the country? Black people.

Our society has created the circumstances in these communities. We decided where it was okay for these issues to persist. In other words, it is not by accident that Black neighborhoods have historically been poor. In the 1960s, as a result of strategic redlining, the poverty rate for Black Americans was over 40 percent. In the 1970s it hovered around 33 percent. Since 2020 it's been closer to 18 percent. The rate has decreased over the past 20 years, but the gap between Black Americans and white ones is still wide. Wherever poverty is prevalent is where crime will thrive, and that includes gun violence. In normal times, there isn't enough work to go around, which can lead people to commit crimes. Regular jobs are hard to find. Jobs that allow people to provide for their families are even harder to find. This is why people start selling drugs and guns, breaking into stores and homes, stealing from cars, taking cars, and engaging in other, more innovative activities made possible by the advancement of technology, such as credit card scamming and fraud.

The kind of deprivation experienced in poor communities is taxing. It spreads through the community and creates desperation, and that desperation leads to animosity. This doesn't mean everyone in the hood is ready to pick up a gun. There are countless hardworking, blue-collar, law-abiding citizens who live in the hood and have lived there for decades. But poverty creates circumstances that encourage someone to color outside the lines, and once they start, it's hard to go back. There are a lot of conflicts as well, driven by gangs that operate in these neighborhoods. Rival drug crews and criminal organizations are always ready to go to war with each other. That hatred goes back generations and, for the most part, is dispersed widely in such communities. All of this leads to nonstop gun violence.

Access to weapons can't be ignored either. Those who don't live in these neighborhoods would be surprised by how easy it is for someone to get their hands on a gun and how frequently people carry them. In normal times they feel like they have to carry a gun for their protection. Access to firearms is not just a problem on the streets of disenfranchised minority neighborhoods, however—it is also an issue in the homes of gun-owning families. If a law-abiding parent has a gun in their house, they're already increasing the likelihood that their child will die as a result of the firearm either by accident or intentionally.

A year in America doesn't go by in which gun ownership isn't a notable issue at some point. It's easy fodder for the media to jump on. People go through stretches where they feel they need to buy more guns, such as around election time when they fear that politicians will come after their firearms. People feel safe when they have their own guns, especially at a time of turmoil.

It's impossible to pinpoint one factor that leads to daily community gun violence. Some of the more consistent factors are poverty, easy access to weapons, and a lack of infrastructure. Now, take these and mix them with the pandemic that began in 2020. In a lot of places, these devastating factors intensified. At first, COVID-19 infections and deaths were disproportionately affecting communities of color (specifically Black people). The death rate for Black Americans as a result of the virus was twice as high as that for white Americans. "We're more vulnerable to this thing," Marvin Bradley, a factory worker in Michigan, said back in 2020 after surviving a COVID infection. He and his wife both got infected in the early months of 2020. His wife, Teresa Bradley, who was a nurse, said that when she was taken through the emergency room after catching the virus, the only other COVID patients she saw were Black. "We know that COVID-19 has disproportionately affected Black and brown communities in terms of hospitalizations and deaths. There was the financial impact of COVID on service sectors and low-income jobs, which have an overrepresentation of Black and brown workers," Dr. Shani Buggs says.

On top of the weight of additional deaths, poor communities essentially became poorer. Many of those who were hanging on to jobs by the skin of their teeth lost them in an instant. The job loss in disenfranchised communities was higher than in the rest of the country. With schools going remote, many kids in these communities were sent home to residences where they didn't have internet or a computer and couldn't log in to attend school. If their parents didn't lose their jobs, it was likely because they had jobs where they had to be in person and couldn't work from home. The threat of homelessness hit people hard. The excessive lack of employment opportunities affected adults and young adults alike and left them without any type of economic security. The lack of access to suitable education, food, and health care increased. Even in neighborhoods that are used to despair, fear was rampant.

"COVID exposed where we have significant gaps in terms of resources, staffing, and the ability to quickly pivot," Dr. Joseph Richardson, a gun violence researcher and professor at the University of Maryland, says. Dr. Richardson also directed a gun violence documentary called *Life after the Gunshot*. "For a long period of time, we've been underfunding and underresourcing programs, so when we had a significant rise in gun violence during COVID, we didn't have enough staffing and resources to respond quickly, efficiently, and effectively to a rising epidemic."

Dr. Richardson is part of a coalition of Black gun violence researchers. As in other professional settings, minorities in the gun violence research space tend to be marginalized and left out of the efforts to secure significant funding and research support. This is why he's worked diligently to come together with other Black gun violence experts and researchers to explore the surge that happened in 2020.

It is already difficult to make a significant impact on poverty as well as gun violence with the community-led social services, summer programs and enrichment programs for kids, food programs for families, and other avenues that are used to address these problems. With the stay-at-home orders putting a halt to much of that work for a significant period of time, the problems were bound to get more severe. Social service workers and violence prevention workers typically deal with people who don't seek outside help. They try to reach the most disconnected groups, which is already hard to do when there isn't a debilitating virus spreading in these communities. All the other city functions slowed down as well. Police departments were affected greatly. Policing slowed down; the court system had to stop. The legal system was suspended for a period.

In addition, many people felt that the government was not prioritizing poor Black neighborhoods when it came to providing supplies and materials to fight the pandemic—things like masks, gloves, hand sanitizer, and equipment for local hospitals. Residents within those communities felt abandoned by their government. "I think everything just added up and led to a lot of frustration, concerns, and anger," Paul Carrillo says.

In the hood areas of Chicago, people on the ground described it as "catching it double" during the month of April 2020. They were dealing with high rates of COVID infections and a high number of shootings. "It's like a double whammy. We have the virus and the violence to worry about," Rodney Phillips, a violence interrupter in Chicago, said at the time. "It's just an uphill battle." Like Roy, Rodney had to be outside on the streets to be effective at his job, but because of the social distancing mandates that were in place, he wasn't able to. Police in the city saw it a bit differently. Authorities said that crime had been ebbing and flowing since the start of the pandemic and they could not confirm how the crisis was affecting violence. They did note that shootings were up in March 2020 compared with March 2019 but that other violent crime was down. This is why the initial mandate from up top was for officers to keep their distance from people and not interact unless it was absolutely necessary. "All you have to do is go on the South Side and you'll see groups of people hanging out and you'll see police parked not doing anything about it," Pastor Corey Brooks, a Chicago community leader, previously said.

The staff at the Brookdale University Hospital Medical Center in Brownsville, Brooklyn, also wasn't prepared. Brookdale is one of the most active hospitals for treating gun violence victims in the area. In the first several months of the pandemic, the staff was grappling with COVID patients and a higher number of gunshot victims. Dr. Dorian Alexander, a member of the Brookdale staff, said in September 2020 that the staff was struggling to save gun-

streets. He knows what's going on. He knows which gangs are beefing, who the shooters are, who the informants are, everything. He'll be the first to tell you he's not involved in anything. He just knows everything. His brother was well regarded in the 1990s, but he's been locked up for over 20 years. His uncle was killed in the early 2000s after he "tried the wrong guy." Tion himself doesn't keep a gun on him, though. He doesn't think he needs it. He grew up in the Tilden projects, and while he doesn't live there anymore, he hangs out there all the time. His thoughts on gun violence in his community? "It's always been like this; no matter what people try, it doesn't change much. I tell kids to just try and get outta here as fast as possible." He hasn't followed his own advice, though. "I got nowhere else to go," he says.

During the summer of 2020, Tion and several gang members stood on a corner near the Van Dyke projects late one night. It was a laid-back gathering for them. They were laughing and drinking. They all had masks but none of them had them on their faces; they were just hanging below their chins.

It was fairly dark out. The only light came from the building they were in front of and the New York City Police Department's mobile floodlight tool that can light up an entire block with bright blue light that to Tion looked white. "Them shits look like the entrance to heaven," one of the gang members said, pointing them out. This night wasn't supposed to be anything special.

So you can imagine their surprise when, out of nowhere, someone shot at them. "It was so quick," Tion says. He didn't get a good look at who the shooter was. In fact, he could barely see where the bullets came from. Tion quickly realized the bullets were for his group, so he took off. His belief now is that it was a rival gang member who spotted the group from across the street and just opened up on them.

He ran off alongside one of the gang members. He heard a few more shots as they ran. The two were in the midst of a dead sprint.

The other gang members must've gone the other way. This wasn't his first time being shot at. "This might've been the seventh or eighth time," he says, but this was the first time he ever took off like that. Usually, he'd duck in such a situation, but for some reason tonight his mind told him to run. Something must've told the gang member next to him to run as well. They ran a good two or three blocks before entering the lobby of one of the public housing complexes. Tion knew the shooter likely wasn't chasing them.

They were gasping for breath in the lobby. Tion had his hands on his knees, bent down. After all, they had been drinking for at least an hour and Tion doesn't spend much time working on his cardio. He wasn't hurt, though, just out of breath. He turned to the gang member.

He had been shot.

A bullet had grazed his shoulder, and he was wiping it and holding it at the same time. He didn't panic, though. This wasn't his first time getting shot, but he was "bleeding like crazy," Tion says. There was blood all over his hand and shoulder. It was late and there was no one in the lobby. "You need an ambulance?" Tion asked, calmly. "Yeah, probably," the gang member responded. As Tion called 911, the gang member took a rag out of his pocket to cover the wound. Tion told the 911 operator that his friend had been shot on the corner, and he gave them the address of the lobby they were in. The operator collected all the information and repeatedly asked how bad it was. Tion downplayed it and said it doesn't look bad and that his friend is up on his feet but he could use some help. "We'll send an ambulance over," the operator said. "They on their way," Tion told his friend. So they waited. And waited and waited and waited. No ambulance. "The fuck taking them so long," Tion said. The gang member just stood there with his hand covering the bullet wound.

Tion's not usually one to deal with the authorities, but he was annoyed so he was about to call them back. "I'm good, this ain't shit," the gang member said. Confused, Tion tried to insist, but because it was just a graze the gang member decided that he'd rather avoid dealing with the police. Tion's seen a lot, but this was a bit surprising. He could understand the logic to some degree but couldn't fathom not going to the hospital for a gunshot wound. As far as he knows, this gang member never went to have a doctor look at it. "He had someone he knows stitch him up," Tion says. The hospitals were so busy, they couldn't respond to a gunshot victim.

The socioeconomic factors that already have a negative impact on gun violence were made worse. As a result, gun violence increased. It's not the sole reason (as previously mentioned, there is no one reason), but most experts, community leaders, and activists who deal with this issue on a daily basis will point to it as a cause of the surge.

Something else happened in 2020: a huge spike in gun purchases. During the first month of the year, many Americans stocked up on firearms. In fact, around 23 million guns were purchased that year, which was a 65 percent increase from 2019. There were also a lot of first-time gun buyers in 2020, over 5 million. Overall, sales went up 40 percent and more than 40 million guns were legally purchased. Because of lapses in data, it's difficult to confirm the exact correlation between legal firearm purchases and the increase in gun violence, but there are some facts that point to a connection.

An increase in the number of legal weapons being purchased also increases the chance they could be funneled into the illegal market. That's what happened in 2020. The Bureau of Alcohol, Tobacco, Firearms and Explosives (ATF) is a federal law enforcement agency that handles illegal firearm trafficking. As a result of tracing nearly 400,000 guns in 2020, the ATF determined that more weapons purchased in 2020 were recovered in crimes in a much shorter time frame than they had been in past years. "People were buying guns like a war was coming," an ATF agent says.

According to the Trace, a nonprofit newsroom that covers gun violence, many of the weapons recovered at crime scenes in 2020 were bought that same year. The ATF collected 87,000 of those types of weapons at crime scenes in 2020. Usually, it takes longer for guns to go from the legal market to the illegal one, but the process ramped up that year. It doesn't help that gun laws in the country are weak to begin with. The increase in gun purchases meant there were more guns inside homes, which leads to more accidental and domestic violence shootings, both of which saw an increase in 2020. The fear that proliferated in 2020 led people to obtain more firearms, whether legally or illegally, which led to more shooting incidents and victims.

In the poor hood neighborhoods, some of the conflicts that already existed got worse. The reason is unclear, and it varies from neighborhood to neighborhood. Community residents and leaders say that social media played a large role in exacerbating the issues between different groups and gangs. "They couldn't get to each other in person for a minute so they started going at each other on social media. I think that set a lot of things off that happened in the summer of 2020," Tamar Manasseh, the founder of Mothers/Men Against Senseless Killings, a Chicago-based anti-violence community organization, says.

Of course, there is no empirical evidence that suggests there's a correlation, but as Tamar points out, there are enough observational examples that highlight the concern. "Folks live their lives online. They share and engage in content that is related to their neighborhood life. So if you live in a neighborhood with high rates of gun violence, a part of what you talk about is what happens in the neighborhood. A large sum of that can be gun violence or gang violence," Dr. Desmond Patton, a professor at the University of Pennsylvania who studies the correlation between social media and gun violence, says. In the case of the pandemic, those gang conflicts were likely relegated to social media at the height of the stay-at-home orders. Since the conflicts got worse in the digital space, they blurred the lines in the physical space. Once people started going back outside, it was on sight.

While there's a certain level of agreement among criminologists and other experts about COVID's impact on gun violence, the issue is complicated and far from settled. "When we think about the effects of the pandemic on gun violence, it most likely did contribute to an increase in gun violence, but truly understanding those effects is quite complex," Professor Rick Rosenfeld explains. "I think it's fair to say the pandemic did not have a straightforward, easily explainable effect on violence. In some ways, I think it curtailed the violence that might have occurred; in other ways it likely exacerbated it. It's really hard to tell which of those influences was stronger," he says. Still, Professor Rosenfeld and others who study these trends believe the pandemic was one of the major contributors to this surge and as more time passes and more analyses are conducted, that direct correlation will become clearer.

No matter what the data say, sometimes the people themselves provide all the context that's needed to explain complexities.

In South Los Angeles, there's a small neighborhood called Vermont Square. It's a two-and-a-half-square-mile community with a population of about 52,000. It's a primarily Latino and Black neighborhood. Like the other South Los Angeles areas, it's a poor neighborhood. Down South Western Avenue, which can be taken all the way to the metropolitan area of Los Angeles, there are a handful of storefronts and businesses along the way—auto parts garages, tire shops, small convenience stores, giant lots, and franchised fast-food restaurants. The homes in residential areas are mostly rentals. They have sizable gaps between them and are not mashed together as in dense inner-city neighborhoods, though this is still considered an urban area.

Kellen grew up in Vermont Square. He lives near the park, which is about six miles south of downtown Los Angeles. His mother is a post office worker and has been for decades. Kellen dabbles in the streets. He's done some "scamming" with a few others in his neighborhood. He's slight and unimposing. He was 17 years old and attending one of the local high schools when the pandemic hit. He and his friends experienced a disconnect as the crisis was unfolding. "We didn't care much about it. We didn't get why everyone was scared," he says. Even when infections started to go up and people were dying, he and his friends weren't that concerned. In March 2020 students were sent home from school and were expected to attend remotely, but Kellen saw this as an opportunity to just hang out. "I didn't do much school after that," he says. His mother was a frontline worker, so he had their home to himself. The pandemic hit Los Angeles County hard the first year. By the end of May 2020, the county was responsible for more than 55 percent of the state's COVID cases and over 3,600 deaths.

During the first few weeks of March 2020, the streets were calm, calmer than Kellen had ever seen them, but that didn't last long. "People were just outside more. You had to really watch your back," he says. The economic stress weighed on the neighborhood. Residents were on edge, and there were fewer police cars driving through. Kellen saw gang conflicts get worse, and he felt that social media played a big part in those disputes. "You couldn't see the nigga you was beefing with face-to-face so you went at him online," he says. Regardless, there were more shootings in Los Angeles and more deaths. Vermont Square had the biggest increase in deaths across the city between January and September 2020 compared with the same time period in 2019. There were 12 homicides in that time period in 2020. In 2019 there were only 3. As a result of what was happening in his neighborhood, Kellen started carrying a gun. Fortunately, he hasn't had to use it, but he feels safer with it. "No one out here is looking out for me," he says. He did end up getting his diploma and is doing "odd jobs" until he figures out his next step. If the pandemic had any impact on his future plans, he's unclear what it was. "I'm not sure where I was headed before it happened," he says.

More than 2,000 miles east of Kellen's neighborhood is Grand Rapids, Michigan, the antithesis of sunny Los Angeles. Though it's the state's second-largest city, the population is fewer than 200,000 people. At first glance, it could appear suburban and quiet, similar to a lot of other midwestern cities. In reality, though, the Black areas in the city struggle with all the socioeconomic issues that plague almost all Black communities. Houses in these neighborhoods look run down or abandoned. The same goes for businesses. Entire blocks look desolate. There's a large liquor store south of the downtown area from which you can see the skyscrapers far out in the distance, signifying how far away the heart of the city is. Next to the liquor store is what looks like an old factory that employed many workers when it operated. East of the liquor store is Joe Taylor Park, where many of the youth spend their free time. The city doesn't look like much but it has its issues, deep-rooted issues.

JD Chapman grew up in the small city. He watched and participated in "the war" happening on the streets as a kid. Drugs and guns were everywhere. Poverty was widespread. JD got into some trouble and spent 10 years in prison. "I think my generation and the generation before me are to blame as far as the streets go. I was born and bred in the streets," JD says. "My generation wasn't able to show the next generation a pathway out of the streets." When he was released at the age of 26, he dedicated his life to showing the youth another path. He runs a local group in the city called Realism Is Loyalty, which works with at-risk kids. The feeling on the ground among community activists is that the city social workers refuse to work with those kinds of youth. "The guys that play with pistols, the guys that are known to stand on the block and sell dope—social services doesn't want to go near them," JD says. The responsibility falls on him and others in the community to prevent the kids from finding themselves in the back of a police car or an ambulance. Before 2020, the city's poor neighborhoods struggled, but gun violence and killings were down. There were just 9 murders in 2018 and 19 in 2019. Once the pandemic started, though, there was an immediate reaction from people in Grand Rapids.

"Everybody was scared, everybody ain't know what was going on. Everything was shut down. Nothing was moving in the city," JD recalls. After the fear came, the crime followed. Property crime went up and auto thefts went "through the roof," JD says. And then came the gun violence. There were over 1,000 gun crimes reported to the police that year and 38 homicides, which was a city record and the highest number since 1993. "The pandemic made things really, really bad because all the resources were sucked out of the hood," JD says.

The group of individuals who weren't afraid during the height of the pandemic in Grand Rapids are the very type of youth whom JD works with. "You couldn't tell young people that COVID was killing people. They think they're invincible," he says. With the schools closed, a lack of supervision, and nothing to do, JD says, the youth were just out in the streets. The community work that JD and others do on the ground in the city requires them to be engaged with the youth on a daily basis. Since 2020, that's been more difficult. He went from seeing the kids one on one multiple times a week to seeing them maybe once a week. JD was usually in constant contact with the schools, families, detention centers, and jails to do his work. All of that came to a halt in 2020. He believes that it greatly contributed to the surge in gun violence. "That first year was bad, man. I never saw the city like that," JD says. He lives near what he considers a new hotspot, which is a gas station around the corner from his home. Before the virus was widespread, this area was already dangerous, but not as dangerous as it became. That gas station could be viewed as a microcosm of what the pandemic represented for poor communities.

Going into 2021, the problems in Grand Rapids persisted, but the homicides themselves dropped back down to 19, which is consistent with some other cities throughout the country. Remember, most homicides in the city and across the country are driven by gun violence. Still, the trends in Grand Rapids reflect the common ebbs and flows of firearm crimes. "Gun violence just has peaks and valleys. The hood economy drives gun violence," JD says.

This has been the case in Grand Rapids since 2020. Homicide numbers went down in 2021 to 19 and then back up in 2022 to 23. These numbers look weak compared with those for larger cities, but since Grand Rapids is so small, the effects of each individual homicide are felt by many people. Almost all of these homicides were done with a firearm. "We just hear a lot of gunfire," JD says.

COVID made this issue worse. There are many people who live in these communities across the country who felt its effects directly. They felt the pain and hopelessness in their neighborhoods get worse. They saw the violence increase with their own eyes. They saw the safety net (which was already flawed) vanish. They saw outlets and venues close down that were there to support the vulnerable and impressionable youth. They saw the hatred escalate. There were people who never thought of owning a gun who either bought one or stole one because they felt they needed protection. And this wasn't just in inner-city communities either; it happened across rural America as well.

Someone who works in corporate America who can do their job from home and who never really had to travel outside their bubble during the worst moments of 2020 probably didn't feel the change. But that's no different from before, when they would never journey into the most poverty-stricken areas and see what life is like for people who live there. No one in these communities wants to live the way they're forced to. There are some people who will shoot others without regard for human life, but that's not the majority. Even those who are involved in the violence know that it's wrong. Black people who live in the hood are not inherently violent and evil. It's the poverty and circumstances that increase the likelihood of someone picking up a gun and using it. The people aren't violent; it's the poverty that's violent.

It's a constant battle. If you're young and you're outside in a lot of these areas, it's hard to avoid the gangs. The circumstances create the violence, and those circumstances got worse in 2020. The disparities that affect minority urban communities make the battle a lot harder. The surge in gun violence happened at different times in different cities. Some spikes started during the lockdowns, some started after. This point can't be stressed enough: there isn't one factor that drives gun violence. Regardless, 2020 was revealing—it brought into stark relief the many elements that together perpetuate the cycle of violence in poor communities.

The pandemic didn't make the communities bad; it just further destabilized the poor structures that already existed in them.

That's one side of what drove the surge in gun violence, but there was another factor as well, something that wasn't anticipated by most, though others were watching it closely the whole time. Law enforcement plays a crucial role in these communities, and that certainly includes what happens around gun violence. It turns out that in the midst of one of the worst public health crises the country and the world had ever faced, another issue was bubbling under the surface. It took a supremely unfortunate event for people to stop what they were doing and pay attention to how law enforcement operates in these communities. What they likely weren't prepared for was how the response to the tragedy would influence gun violence.

3

Defund

It's a few days into June 2020 in Crown Heights, Brooklyn. The pandemic is in full swing and Roy is still wearing multiple hats as he continues his violence prevention work and helps on the front lines with the spread of COVID-19. At this moment, however, people in the neighborhood aren't focused on a virus. There's a lot of tension on the streets, which is in part a response to the tragic death of George Floyd in Minneapolis nearly two weeks ago as a result of the action of a city police officer. The killing hasn't just sparked a visceral reaction in Minneapolis; people all over the country are angry. But the current concern among those in Crown Heights is also a response to another Black man's encounter with the police.

On the night of June 2, NYPD officers responded to a signal from ShotSpotter, which is a popular and controversial device that law enforcement uses to detect gunshot incidents. The alert came from the corner of Bergen Street and Rochester Avenue, right by the Kingsborough Houses. This public housing complex takes up the entire block, with 16 buildings in total. All of them are around six stories tall and have thousands of apartment units. The police aren't unfamiliar with this area, as a lot of shootings happen there.

Residents are so used to gunshots, especially in the summer months, that they barely bat an eye at them. When the officers got to the scene, it was quiet and dark. Some people were out and around the complex, but nothing looked out of the ordinary. People weren't scrambling or ducking for cover, which led the police to believe that the worst part of the incident was over. In a courtyard within the complex, the cops found a man, Terrance Colclough, wounded from a gunshot. He was hit in the leg and told the cops that the shooter had to be nearby. They quickly went looking for him. One of the officers found someone on his knees behind a tree. The man, Malik Tyquan Graves, seemed to be hiding. The officer asked if he had heard any gunshots. When Malik looked up, the officer quickly said "stop" multiple times. He saw the gun on Malik's lap. This was the shooter.

The officer pulled his gun out and yelled, "Put it down," to Malik, who now had his own gun in his hand. The cop repeated the command several times. "Put it down!" he yelled. Other officers arrived, and they yelled at Malik too. "Yo!" "Drop the gun!" "Drop the fucking gun, bro!" "Drop it and move!" It was like a scene out of a gritty cop drama. The officer who was closest to Malik started to back up, with his weapon still pointed at him. Other officers were behind parked cars in the street with their guns out too. They all continued to yell at him. At this point, it was not just the police yelling at Malik to put the gun down; nearby residents were too. One said, "It's not worth it, bro!" Malik stood up, with the gun still in his hands. Now the community and the police in unison were begging and pleading with Malik to drop the gun. Everyone knew where this was going to end up, and it sounded like no one wanted it to go that way. Not the cops and not the residents. The warnings from the police and pleas from residents went on for over two minutes but Malik never dropped the gun. The yells turned into a din, just a prolonged series of loud noises. Then there was a lull, a short, quiet moment. This could end with him just dropping the gun and getting arrested. He already shot someone, but no one needed to die. All he had to do was put the gun down.

Then *pap, pap, pap, pap, pap, pap, pap, pap, pap!*

The cops pulled their triggers. It was quick and resembled a firing squad. Residents who were watching ducked down, either in their apartments or outside by a car or tree. In total, 62 bullets were fired at Malik and 12 of them hit him. Ten officers shot at him. "It felt like everyone on the block was screaming at him. I don't think those cops really wanted to shoot him," one resident who watched the incident says. Malik died at a nearby hospital. The police later said the weapon that he had was out of bullets. While the loss of anyone to gun violence is a tragedy for a community, this shooting was justified from a law enforcement perspective. Malik's mother didn't feel that way. "It was overkill—too many bullets and too many cops," Motique Graves previously said. "They didn't give my son a chance. He was no threat to them. He didn't point no gun at them."

Roy was hurt when he heard about this incident. It felt like it was compounding an already painful time for the community. He got in touch with the mother of Malik's child to offer any support he could. He also attended a vigil and protest on June 6, 2020, outside the Kingsborough projects. Roy went as a community member, not as a violence interrupter. "I don't know if I even went there expecting anything. It was just a lot that was going on and I wanted to show my support." This protest was a peaceful one, which hadn't always been the case that summer.

By this point in 2020, everyone was familiar with the phrase "defund the police." It was being shouted at protests across the country, journalists were writing about it, cable news anchors were debating it, politicians were trying to figure out if they could actually do it, and, of course, law enforcement was grappling with it. There were also protests against the police happening all across the country. Many of them were peaceful but a lot of them weren't.

In July, Roy and his organization put together a march against gun violence in the community. That summer, shootings and murders were drastically increasing across the city. The march wasn't supposed to be about the police. As a violence prevention organization, they tried to stay out of the policing issue. "While we were all deeply saddened by those events on a personal level, as an organization, we never took a stance on that," he stresses.

During this July event, some local elected officials spoke. The politicians did talk about community violence, but it was in the context of urging residents not to kill each other when there was another group, the police, already killing them. Some of the speakers were also pushing the idea of defunding the police with the goal of eventually abolishing them. This was what some politicians were advocating for at the time. It's taboo to bring this up, but if you ask those who actually live in the communities that have to deal with gun violence on a daily basis, they will say that the effects of the defund movement didn't help this problem. To many, it made it worse.

When George Floyd entered Cup Foods, a convenience store on the south side of Minneapolis, on May 25, he was already having a rough year. In January he lost his delivery driving job. In March the club he did security at closed. That same month, he was hospitalized for a drug overdose. The next month he caught COVID. On the day he died, he was buying a pack of cigarettes. A store employee believed that Floyd had used a fake $20 bill and called the police. What happened afterward reflects the fear and uneasiness that a lot of Black people have when it comes to police interactions. There has always been a great deal of tension between the Black community and the police who operate in their neighborhoods. Many trace this back to the days of slavery, but you don't have to go that far back. Whether it's in the context of something routine like a traffic stop or a harmless inquiry, Black people, specifically Black men, are usually viewed as a threat. If you're a police officer and you work in a poor Black neighborhood, most of the criminals you apprehend are Black men. Officers are often conditioned to view most of the Black men they come across as a threat.

In the case of George Floyd, he was first approached by two officers—J. Alexander Kueng and Thomas Lane. They asked him several times to show his hands. There was a struggle when Floyd got out of his car. They suspected he was "on something," but Floyd told them he was just scared. It turns out he had significant levels of fentanyl in his body. Another struggle occurred when the officers tried to put him in their car. He told them he was dealing with anxiety and claustrophobia. Two more officers came, Tou Thao and Derek Chauvin, the latter of whom was the highest-ranking officer among the four.

After Chauvin arrived, there was another struggle while Floyd was in the backseat of the police car. He was pulled out and placed face down on the pavement. Then three of the officers tried to hold him down. Kueng held his torso and Lane had his legs pressed down, but it was Chauvin who took it a step further.

Chauvin had his knee pressed against Floyd's neck. Onlookers were filming at this point. Some of them yelled at Chauvin to stop. At the same time, Floyd was begging for his life. "I can't breathe!" "I'm about to die!" "Mama!" "Please, the knee in my neck, I can't breathe!" It wasn't just the actions of Chauvin that would grasp the nation, it was the level of indifference expressed on his face. It went past being evil or sinister. That requires emotion. There was no emotion coming from him.

He looked like he did not care about Floyd's life.

He also looked like he didn't care that people were watching him. There was a level of arrogance emanating from his face, like, "I'm law enforcement and I can do what I want." Chauvin knelt on Floyd's neck for over eight minutes until an ambulance arrived. Floyd was taken to the hospital and pronounced dead about an hour later. Once the videos circulated online, everything changed.

Typically, when a high-profile police killing of a Black citizen happens, the reaction follows a pattern: outrage, protesting, the investigation into the incident, some policy changes within the department, an outside investigation of the department, and finally an announcement that the officers didn't do anything wrong and won't be charged criminally. In some cases, the federal government will do an internal investigation or review of the department, and if it finds patterns of abuse or misconduct, the department will be placed under a consent decree. This is a mandate that ensures that the department makes changes in line with constitutional protections. Minneapolis was no stranger to controversy in its police department. Its history of discrimination, misconduct, and abuse is well documented. Any Black person in 2020 could tell you that this one felt different. It could have been how gut-wrenching the video was; it could have been the fact that, even in the midst of a deadly virus that was disproportionately affecting Black people, they still had to deal with the threat of violence at the hands of the police for something as minuscule as an allegedly counterfeit $20 bill. Whatever it might have been, to see and hear a 46-year-old man begging for his mother in his final moments was too much. Sandra Richardson, a Minneapolis activist who was raised five blocks away from where Floyd was killed, watched the video in horror. "It wasn't even like there was a human being under [Chauvin's knee]. That incident lit a match in the community," she says.

So the city erupted into protests. The protesting started peacefully, but it didn't take long for it to become chaotic and violent. In Minneapolis, property was destroyed, including the Third Precinct building, which is two miles east of where Floyd was killed. The city saw looting, violent confrontations with the police, and a large number of arrests. The protests didn't stop there; they spread to cities all across the country—Los Angeles, New York, Atlanta, and Washington, DC, among other locations. These other places didn't get as bad as Minneapolis did, but there was still loot-ing and violence. What followed was one of the largest series of civil rights protests in American history. It came with a price, though. The total financial cost of the damages across the country eclipsed $1 billion. "The relationship with the police was already in a critical form, but that summer it just totally deteriorated. People just lost regard and respect for the police," Tyrone Parker, a founding member of the Alliance of Concerned Men in Washing-ton, DC, says. It went beyond justice for Floyd. Surprisingly, it seemed like his family might get that after all four officers in-volved were fired and criminally charged. From the perspective of the protesters, this was about change, widespread change, but the calls were for more than "criminal justice reform."

The idea of defunding the police was not new. *The End of Polic-ing*, written by Brooklyn College professor Alex S. Vitale in 2017, could be viewed as a benchmark for the calls activists made in 2020. The book argues that simple reform of the police is not enough and that the goal should be to eventually get to a place where the police can be abolished. So this proposal didn't come out of nowhere, it just hadn't hit the mainstream consciousness of the country. The summer of 2020 changed that. The Black Vi-sions Collective, a nonprofit community-based organization in Minneapolis, was the first group to popularize the term "defund the police" after Floyd's murder. Once the term caught on, many activists across the country started to use it.

The phrase, however, is used with a variety of intentions. The most accepted definition of "to defund" is to divest funds from po-lice departments and put that money into more community-led programs and nonpolice forms of addressing public safety like ed-ucation, housing, youth services, social services, violence pre-vention, mental health services, homelessness outreach, and other types of programs. There were others who used "to defund" to mean to abolish the police entirely. Some believe a new form of public safety should be created after departments get abolished, while others believe that the focus should solely be on community, grassroots, and social service organizations and that there shouldn't be any form of law enforcement in the picture.

Police departments have not been defunded, though. Not in any significant way. Shortly after Floyd's murder and the protests that followed, a majority of the city council in Minneapolis promised to dismantle the police department and create a new public safety department. They didn't follow through on that. Some councilmembers walked back their initial comments; others had different interpretations of what defunding actually meant, indicative of the issues with the term. During the November 2021 city elections, there was a ballot question asking if voters wanted to replace the police with a new department of public safety. Fifty-six percent of them said no.

The reality is that most of the large city police departments either left their budgets the same or increased them going into 2021. New York City and Los Angeles made some significant cuts to their police department funds, with city leaders in New York slashing $1 billion from the $6 billion police budget in 2021. But the number in New York rose again the next year. The police budget in 2021 was $5.2 billion, and in 2022 it was $5.4 billion. Nationwide, police funding increased in 2022. The US spending on police would rank higher than what other countries spend on their military budgets. But while the movement to defund the police does not seem to have had a significant effect on police budgets, some believe that it has actually had a negative effect on the communities hit the hardest by police violence.

Baltimore is a poster child for everything that's wrong with the criminal justice system in the United States. Gun violence, police corruption, mass incarceration, the war on drugs—the city has dealt with it all. "We didn't get here overnight. These problems are deeply rooted in systemic challenges in this city," Baltimore mayor

Brandon Scott says. Before Freddie Gray died while in police custody in 2015, community leaders on the west side of Baltimore, which is notorious for its struggles with crime, were celebrating because they had their lowest number of homicides in over a decade. "The trajectory of violence in Baltimore City did a complete 180 shift when the Freddie Gray death happened," Ray Kelly, a community leader in West Baltimore, says. Ray is the executive director of the Citizens Policing Project, a grassroots organization that helps community members have a say in the policies and practices of the police in their area. After Gray's controversial death—and the civil unrest that followed—shootings and killings went up in the city. "Our numbers have been consistent since the riots and the unrest following Freddie Gray's death," Ray points out.

This was also the case in Ferguson after Michael Brown was killed by a cop in 2014. The city was rocked by protests and unrest, followed by a surge in gun violence, a pattern that is now known in criminal justice circles as "the Ferguson effect." Chicago experienced the same thing after Laquan McDonald was killed by police in 2014. The same thing happened in Minneapolis after Floyd was killed, and in Philadelphia after police officers shot and killed Walter Wallace Jr. in the fall of 2020. There's a clear pattern here. "When we have these very high-profile instances of police brutality, we see these surges in gun violence," Dr. Shani Buggs says. "I don't know that we truly understand what the phenomenon is, but it does exist."

So what happened in these cities? There is a belief among certain community members, leaders, and experts that the police stopped being proactive and pulled back—they started depolicing. There has been evidence of this over the last several years, especially in Baltimore after Gray was killed. "Literally overnight our rates of shootings and homicides went up like 70 percent," Professor Daniel Webster, who's based in Baltimore, says. "The police stopped doing their jobs in certain areas." Ray saw this firsthand. "The violence was escalating and it's been going unchecked since Gray was killed," he says. Baltimore is in a unique position because it was one of the only cities in 2020 that did not see a drastic increase in homicides from 2019. For it, that increase had happened five years earlier after Gray's death. The city's police stopped doing the things that actually help a poor community: solving violent crimes and targeting known violent criminals.

David Simon, the creator of *The Wire*, which is viewed by many as the greatest television show of all time, is also supremely familiar with the streets of Baltimore. Much of his career as a journalist and as a TV writer has explored the decaying dynamics of the city from the law enforcement side and the community side. Today he still lives there and is not shy about his thoughts on how policing has affected what's happened in his city. "The great argument among people who either believe all cops are bastards, or defund the police, and people who say back the blue is horseshit," David says. "Neither one of them are admitting to a couple of equivocations, that our communities in Baltimore are overpoliced and underpoliced at the same time." Simon's latest Baltimore TV project, *We Own This City*, covers the rise and fall of the rogue Gun Trace Task Force, which wreaked havoc on community members in the city. That miniseries explicitly makes the connection between a work stoppage among police as a result of the Freddie Gray unrest and the rise in gun violence that followed.

This is what Minneapolis community members saw happen in their city as well. They believe that the mass protesting and calls for defunding led police officers to revolt. "I used to see cops on my block all the time. That stopped in the summer of 2020," one elderly South Minneapolis resident says. As large scale as the Freddie Gray and Michael Brown incidents were, they didn't touch the level of impact George Floyd's death did. People who had never set foot in Minneapolis were protesting in their own cities, disparaging the police, calling them useless, telling them they weren't needed. "You can only hear that so much until you react to it," a homicide detective in Minneapolis explains. "Police are human beings too, so many of us were offended by those proclamations and some reacted in an emotional and unprofessional manner."

Police officers felt this way across the country. About 337 miles east of Minneapolis is Milwaukee, another small city whose police department has a checkered past. Between 2010 and 2020 the city spent over $40 million on police brutality cases. Like almost every other major city, Milwaukee saw its murders go up in 2020. The circumstances of the pandemic were a factor, but as law enforcement sees it, the violence was a by-product of what happened nationally with policing. "There was a lot of animus toward law enforcement. Police legitimacy was in question," Paul Formolo, the assistant chief of police in the city, says. A Philadelphia police captain agrees and says a lot of officers were offended by the things that were being said. "This prompted a slowdown in productivity by some of these police officers, and I strongly believe that the criminal element picked up on that. They picked up on the slowdown," the captain says.

Todd Morris, a police officer in Brooklyn, experienced all the turmoil in the summer of 2020. He sees both sides of it. Todd is a neighborhood coordinating officer (NCO). NCOs are supposed to build a relationship with the communities that they police. There are 77 NYPD precincts across New York City, and each precinct has between four and five NCOs. "For me, it was an honor to be part of this program. The department heard the concerns from people [about not having a real connection with law enforcement] and we responded to that," he says. He operates in what could be considered a dangerous area of Brooklyn. He and his other NCO officers had spent the last few years making headway in developing a connection with their communities. "Residents can call us about anything at all. We want them to call us about the small things. That's how you build rapport."

But he feels some of that headway was damaged in the summer of 2020. When the unrest happened in Brooklyn, the police were being watched closely. Todd felt a bit more hostility during this period. He got fewer calls from residents even though there was more going on. Many of his colleagues were offended by the rhetoric spreading, he says. Some of them even felt vindicated when gun violence increased as the summer went on. "They looked at it as proof that we're needed," he says with some shame. He doesn't believe a real work stoppage happened; he thinks people weren't calling the police as much.

Others in Brooklyn aren't buying that the police didn't take a step back, though, especially members of a violence prevention organization in Brooklyn called Save Our Streets (SOS). They were on the front lines in 2020. They say that when the calls for defunding started and city leaders—like violence interrupters and credible messengers—began touting other ways to address public safety, the police stopped going the "extra mile" to do their jobs. The SOS members in Bed-Stuy say the police even asked them to take a stand against the protesting that was going on, something they did not agree to do. "We denounce all gun violence. Now the police have a job to do. If they shoot someone because they had a gun, then that was their job," Joshua Simon, a violence interrupter with SOS Bed-Stuy, says. "We won't do a shooting response to that, but we [are] not going to get out there and praise that. There was no way in the world we were going out there to stand with [the police]."

A work stoppage is hard to prove, and it's hard to prove what kind of impact it had on gun violence. Anecdotally, there are a lot of reports that police were instructed by their command to do less policing in the streets during the summer of 2020. "You definitely have seen more depolicing in cities and police not actively engaging in proactive policing, and that could be backlash from George Floyd," Dr. Joseph Richardson says. What is verifiable is that many departments have struggled to retain officers. Since the summer of 2020, major police agencies across the country have dealt with staff shortages and open positions. This has made it more difficult for the departments to be proactive in their efforts to address violent crime. Another wrinkle from the chaos of 2020 was the tension that arose between certain district attorneys' offices and police departments. Some departments feel like there are prosecutors who are moving toward deincarceration so they're unwilling to prosecute some violent crimes, including gun offenses. From the police perspective, it's difficult to be proactive when you know that your state's attorney's office might not prosecute a case you bring them. "Some of these [district attorney's] offices and police departments are not speaking the same language," Dr. Richardson says. "You have tension with what the DA offices see as their role and what the police see as their role." This is the case in a handful of cities, including Philadelphia and Baltimore. The police feel like they don't have support from prosecutors.

All in all, the chaos that follows a high-profile police killing is usually isolated to the city where the shooting occurred, but the ramifications of Floyd's murder reached many other areas in the summer of 2020. The emotional response from community members who actually live in the areas where these police killings happen is not baseless. How could it be? These are people who live in constant despair and feel betrayed and forgotten by city leaders. Their feelings are rooted in decades of racism and discrimination at the hands of the government, including the police. Do you think $40 million over 10 years for police brutality cases in Milwaukee is bad? How about $67 million for police misconduct in Chicago in 2021 alone? New York City reached that same number more than halfway through 2022 for lawsuits against the

NYPD. The numbers don't fully represent all the brutality and misconduct that goes on, but they highlight how costly all of this is. The Floyd incident happened at a time when many communities were overwhelmed and people felt let down by their government. While dealing with that, they also still had to deal with the possibility of a cop killing them for a nonviolent crime.

Before the defund movement emerged, law enforcement across the country already had trouble addressing inner-city gun crimes. The numbers before 2020 were on the decline, but remember it's a constant issue in the hood. Police have trouble taking proactive measures against gun violence, and a lot of their work is reactive. People are either afraid or unwilling to tell the police what is going on. They rarely have witnesses come forward. If there's a conflict going on, those involved aren't going to the police; they'd rather handle it themselves. For the most part, the police don't have a good relationship with the neighborhoods they patrol. This goes back to the 1990s and how the war on drugs changed what was considered good policing. There are plenty of instances of daily misconduct happening in these city police departments that only people in the neighborhood know about—instances of police misconduct, brutality, or violence that don't lead to a high-profile death or a payout to the family. It's not just horrible situations like the Gun Trace Task Force scandal in Baltimore. It can be simple, routine misconduct, and it is not just individuals who engage in it; it's entire departments. All of this increases gun violence. "I can't blame folks for not having faith in the police," Paul Carrillo explains.

Incidents like what happened to Tyre Nichols in Memphis are exactly what make community members believe that it's a systemic issue within entire police departments. In early January 2023, Nichols—23 and Black—was on his way home when he was stopped by five Memphis police officers. These officers were part of an elite anticrime unit known as Street Crimes Operation to Restore Peace in Our Neighborhoods, or SCORPION. The officers stopped him for "reckless driving" and pulled him out of the car. They told the young man to get on the ground and threatened to tase him. Confused, he told them he didn't do anything, but they didn't care. They pushed him to the ground and again threatened to tase him. The threats and commands continued until Nichols was able to get free and run. The officers eventually caught him and got him to the ground again.

They began punching him, kicking him, and beating him with batons. It was constant and relentless. Nichols was defenseless on the ground and called out for help. At one point he called out for his mother. He didn't hit them back, not once. After the cops beat him into a daze, they sat him up against one of the police cars. One of the officers, summing up their actions, simply said, "I was straight hitting him with haymakers, dog." Nichols died a few days later from his injuries.

All five officers were fired and charged. They were charged with multiple crimes, including second-degree murder. The SCORPION unit was disbanded by Memphis police chief Cerelyn J. Davis. As it turns out, Chief Davis had created the unit, which was similar to a unit she commanded in Atlanta called Run Every Drug Dealer Out of Georgia, or REDDOG. That unit was disbanded in 2011 after a series of high-profile incidents of excessive force involving its members.

What the SCORPION unit did is exactly what police are not supposed to do, as any law enforcement official who watched the body-camera footage of the incident will tell you. But among the people in communities that have to deal with such units, the perception is that this is what all police do. That, in turn, has a negative impact on policing, which affects how they're able to protect communities from gun violence.

It's not just about how often the police kill an unarmed Black person, because that is a statistically rare occurrence. Since at least the early 2010s, police have killed around 1,000 people a year. While Black men are (not surprisingly) at a much higher risk of being killed by the police than anyone else in the country, police shooting deaths make up less than 2 percent of all the shooting deaths each year. By the time Baltimore reached 250 homicides in 2022, just one of them was from a cop killing a citizen. The data on police killings are flawed and difficult to track nationally because of how each individual law enforcement agency—there are 18,000 across the country—gathers and puts out its crime stats. There are some national independent databases that try to collect this information, but the earliest they go back is 2013. It's likely that the police killed a lot more people in the 1970s than they do today.

Still, overly aggressive policing has had a disastrous effect on generations of low-income citizens. Look at all the agencies that the Department of Justice investigated for bad conduct. These probes usually reveal disturbing patterns of discrimination against Black people and other civil rights violations. That bad policing contributes to a rise in violent crime because it creates more mistrust in these communities. A city like Baltimore has trouble filling a jury for murder trials because enough regular citizens don't trust what a cop has to say. That's a direct result of bad policing. Now, there are plenty of situations that call for police to use force and violence. Sometimes they have to shoot and kill someone and it's completely justified. After all, they're paid to protect people from crime and violence. The protests and calls to action are in response to unlawful police violence. Officers, sergeants, captains, and chiefs are all aware of what the difference is. Unlawful police violence leads to community violence.

Does that mean residents who live in neighborhoods that hear gunshots day in and day out don't want the police in their communities? Absolutely not. An August 2020 Gallup poll showed that 81 percent of Black Americans want the same level of policing or more of it. A 2022 study by Pew Research shows violence and crime as the number one concern for Black adults. Go to any community board meeting at a police precinct in the hood and you'll hear loud and clear what Black people in those communities are concerned about. "Where are the goddamn cops?! We need them," one Black woman said during a Brownsville community board meeting, prompting applause. When the defund movement took off in the summer of 2020, some of the loudest voices didn't represent the struggling communities. Many of the residents in these neighborhoods believe that the young activists who made the most noise during the height of the defund movement in 2020 didn't actually live in the affected areas. "All the defund the police stuff was really coming from privileged white suburban kids," Kathryn Bocanegra, who does a lot of outreach work on gun violence in Chicago, says. "I've been working with families of homicide victims since 2007. I have never once heard a family of a homicide victim say they don't want police to be a part of their life."

If you talk to enough people who live and work in poor minority neighborhoods, you'll find they feel that the activists who were advocating for defunding the police didn't speak for folks in the hood. In fact, some believe that certain activists used the tragedy of George Floyd and the mayhem that followed it for their own agendas and weren't really concerned about how it would affect the neighborhoods directly. "We're just pawns, man. Our neighborhoods are just used for politics. You think those people actually care about [unlawful police violence]? That was just a hot issue to jump on [in 2020]," Tion, the Brownsville resident whose friend was grazed by a bullet in 2020, says. Even those who don't live in those communities could see it. Professor Webster says the movement was "fracturing an already tenuous relationship between police and communities most impacted by violence."

There are also political implications to this. The defund movement has been aligned with Democrats and progressives, even though they've tried to distance themselves from the movement. As previously stated, defunding means different things to different people, and those who use it to mean abolishing the police have created an atmosphere where politicians who may be more moderate Democrats can't advocate for anything on the policing side because they'll be attacked. "The abolitionist movement has little affirmative guidance on what leaders should do in response to gun violence," Thomas Abt says. "If defund was just a way of saying 'be bold' in terms of justice reform, I'd happily engage in that conversation. The problem is that the actual language of abolitionism inhibits that discussion." The anti-cop rhetoric and the idea of being completely against the policing system do not reflect the stance of people who live in neighborhoods that struggle with gun violence.

This doesn't mean people in the hood don't support the idea of reallocating police funds. Many people want to see investment in social services and other community-led alternatives to the police. The few who aren't opposed to abolishment look at it as something that can happen down the road when (or if) all the other inequalities in their communities are dealt with. Until then, they know the police are necessary. Protests and rallies against police misconduct and unlawful police violence in the hood should not be misconstrued as indications that those communities support the defunding or abolishment of police departments.

There were certainly people shouting and protesting in Atlanta when everything blew up in 2020. For at least the last 20 years, the metropolitan area of Atlanta has been a popular spot in the South. This is thanks in part to the weather, the locale, and the city's place in hip-hop culture. It's a nice small city to live in. In the last several years, it's been viewed as the "Hollywood of the South." Tyler Perry, a prolific and noteworthy filmmaker, has a 330-acre studio space in southwest Atlanta, which contributes to the city's economy. But anguish exists on the fringes of the downtown area.

Whether it's the east side or the west side, you'll find abandoned and rundown houses. The housing project complexes look like they're from another time period. They are rife with cracked and broken windows, and some have boards where windows are supposed to be. They're falling apart as if they haven't been renovated once since they were built. Some of the housing projects are being demolished as well. Homeless people hang out under the bridges. Gas stations are plenty. Bullets holes are easy to spot in the windows and doors of these stations. Davante Griffin, who is local to the area, says, "There's always a shooting at gas stations." Even with a few updates and clear signs of gentrification, much of Atlanta is plagued by poverty and violence.

"I've had someone come to me and say they'd kill someone I was having an issue with for $250," Davante says.

When the pandemic started, people in Atlanta weren't feeling it the same way it was felt in other places across the country. The city never really shut down the way other cities did. In the hood, though, once some of the relief money started coming through and was reaching certain people's pockets, conflicts arose. "The people who wasn't getting the relief money was mad at the people who were getting it. There was a lot of hating going on," Davante explains, adding that this led to more confrontations and shootings. To other Atlanta residents, though, that's nothing new.

"How I've lived and grown up, gun violence has always been a constant in Atlanta," says Joshua Byrd, who leads anti–gun violence efforts for 100 Black Men of Atlanta, a coalition of Black men who work to address some of the most pressing issues in the city. He's also a professor, security consultant, retired Marine, and former deputy sheriff in DeKalb County, Georgia. Joshua is sturdy and polished. Around 5 feet 10, he has a real professional presence about him. His family has deep roots in Atlanta: they've been there since 1867. He's not a stranger to the gun crimes that go on either. He saw someone get killed when he was 7.

Nearly three weeks after Floyd was murdered, Rayshard Brooks, a 27-year-old Black man, was confronted by two Atlanta police officers when he fell asleep in a car blocking a Wendy's drive-through. After a very cordial and respectful conversation between Brooks and the officers, the situation took a serious turn when the officers attempted to arrest Brooks. He was able to get one of their tasers and tried to run away. One of the cops, Garrett Rolfe, chased Brooks. As he was running, Brooks fired the taser at Rolfe, who took his gun out and shot at him three times. Brooks was hit twice. He later died. The entire incident was captured by body-camera footage.

To no one's surprise at the time, people took to the streets in protest. The Wendy's was set on fire. Police and protesters went at each other. Some of the demonstrators were arrested. In a truly unfortunate event, an 8-year-old girl was shot and killed when her car was shot at by a protester on July 4, 2020. Today the Wendy's is gone, demolished shortly after the death of Brooks. The area where the restaurant used to be is surrounded by dozens of memorials to Brooks. Joshua says the police have always had a poor relationship with the Black community in the city, but it was made worse after the murders of Floyd and Brooks. The community in Atlanta was less trusting of the police, but at the same time, the police in Atlanta made their feelings about the incident very clear.

Just a day after Brooks's death, Officer Rolfe was fired, and a few days after that he was charged with murder. The other officer involved, Devin Brosnan, was charged with aggravated assault. The day after Rolfe was charged, officers in the department held a series of mass strikes in the form of "blue flu" protesting, which is when officers use their sick days in solidarity and do not report to work. Nearly 200 officers did not work for four days, from June 17 to June 20. Police were not responding to calls in a handful of areas. During this stretch, arrests were down over 70 percent.

When police don't answer calls, people don't know where to turn, especially in poor neighborhoods. "You can't call 311 when they shooting up the block," one Atlanta resident says. Even though the strike by the Atlanta Police Department was mostly in the immediate aftermath of Brooks's death, residents say it's had a lingering effect on crime. Joshua had a nephew who was shot in the leg over the summer of 2022, and a friend of the nephew was killed during this incident. "I mean, they lit him up. He was unrecognizable," Joshua says. The police were very slow to respond. "It was over an hour," Joshua says, still in disbelief. "The slow response time leads to [people] feeling like they have to handle things on their own because they know the police aren't coming."

In Joshua's eyes, people who support defunding aren't thinking about these factors. "You've got different camps of defund the police. You've got the liberal defund the police, who are really talking about how you could abolish the police, and you got the more conservative people who say they want to reallocate funds from the police," Joshua says. His understanding of people who live in the hood is similar to what others have said about the movement: "I keep my ear pretty close to the streets. I don't know anybody that wants to defund the police." It's not that the police aren't responding or aren't putting the extra effort into protecting civilians citywide; it's just in the hood areas where Black people live. As far as people in the city are concerned, the summer of 2020 did no favors for the community's relationship with the police or for the day-to-day shootings. By 2022, both officers in Brooks's case had been cleared of charges.

Like every other factor that affects gun violence, you can't completely blame the defund movement for the 2020 surge, just as you can't completely blame the pandemic. But the movement can't be disassociated from the violent surge that followed either. Again, this movement did not come out of nowhere. It was bubbling for decades across the country. When George Floyd was killed and the national movement began, no one from Minneapolis was surprised it started there. Local activists and community leaders in the city had been fighting for reforms in the department for decades. They tried to plead their case in press conferences, city council meetings, and state legislature sessions. "The reality is that our city and elected officials were warned several years ago that this was likely to happen if they did not rein in the Minneapolis police department and also address the economic inequality that African-Americans here face," Nekima Levy Armstrong, a civil rights attorney and founder of the Racial Justice Network in Minneapolis, previously said. "They failed to take action and so this is really the outcome of that."

Those circumstances can be seen in pretty much every major city with a sizable Black population and a flawed police department. A death at the hands of a police officer is often the final straw. There are plenty of other occurrences before the death that lead to animosity between the community and the police—unauthorized stops and searches, unauthorized home searches, harassment, unjust arrests, disrespectful treatment, not responding to calls, and so on. If cops across the board treated people in the hood the way they treat people in affluent white neighborhoods, there would be no demands to defund the police. It would also help if meaningful legislation were passed, like the George Floyd Justice in Policing Act that was introduced in 2021. The bill was intended to address racial bias, abuse of power, and misconduct in policing, but it couldn't pass the Senate.

The defund movement wasn't some con that people devised to stir up trouble in poor neighborhoods; it was the manifestation of real concerns. Still, it was misguided. The police are not going anywhere anytime soon. Everyone knows this. Cities will not abolish their police departments, and the few cities that tried didn't follow through on it. It would be nice if cities like Los Angeles, New York, and Chicago could take some of the funds from their inflated police budgets and put them into social services and other community-led programs. That would help address some of the inequalities, which, in turn, would address gun violence. Aside from such adjustments, though, police department budgets likely aren't going to be touched much as long as police are needed.

The fact remains that police are needed in poor Black communities to combat violent crime, specifically gun crimes. They need to be part of the solution. "Public safety goes beyond the police, but the police play a significant role in this too," Mayor Brandon Scott says. There is no scenario in which they won't be part of the solution, so the best thing to do is to find a way for them to be effective while doing the least harm. Fortunately, that's possible.

PART II

The Sustained Solutions

4

Strategic Policing

Roy remembers the first time he ever saw a police officer. When he was a kid, his uncle passed away after a bout with cancer. He died in the house, surrounded by his family. Paramedics showed up, and alongside them were a couple of police officers. The first thing he noticed were their guns. He kept pointing at them and alerting his grandmother that they were armed, though his grandmother told him it was okay, that the cops were there to help them, not hurt them. Because Roy grew up on a block that was very community oriented and tight-knit, the adults had a relationship with cops who walked the beat in front of their houses. "They would give us candy when we were trick-or-treating. We would take pictures with them," Roy explains.

That all changed when he became a teenager. He skipped school and would get chased by the cops. They became the enemy and he wanted to avoid them at all costs. "I developed this perception that it's us versus them and the goal was to not get caught by them," Roy says. When his street activities really heated up, he had to abide by a code: no interactions with the police whatsoever, unless you were arrested.

Well, that happened—Roy was arrested plenty of times before he eventually went to prison. On one particular occasion in 1991, Roy got arrested for a robbery that the police thought he did. They took him right off the streets near his apartment building and brought him to the 75th Precinct in East New York. Not only was the neighborhood notorious for its crime, but the precinct itself was infamous for the levels of corruption officers engaged in. In the 1990s, the East New York neighborhood was known as New York City's killing field. When Roy walked into the building it was a madhouse. Cops everywhere, phones ringing, nonstop movement, men locked up in the holding cell. It was musky inside, as if a window hadn't been opened all day.

The officers had him sit down at a desk. The chair was wooden and uncomfortable. He kept squirming around. The station had bright fluorescent lights. The cops—two white officers—had no intention of being friendly. It was like they wanted him to be scared, to be intimidated. And he certainly was. Despite his rep on the streets, here he was just another Black guy in a police station. He took note of all the Black men in the holding cells. "These guys looked like they lived hard lives," he says. Roy knew if he said the wrong thing, he'd be right there in one of those cells. The two officers explained that he was a suspect in an armed robbery incident that happened on the streets in early October. "You're the guy. Your name is Martel, right?" one of the officers asked him. Roy said no and that he wasn't the person they were looking for. Coincidentally, Roy was already in the system for a weapons charge from earlier in the month and had been released while the case was pending.

Roy was a full-blown stickup kid at this point, but he was not involved in this particular robbery. He knew he couldn't really be mad at the police for putting a different robbery on him, though. "It's not like I can tell them I didn't do this one but I've done other ones," Roy points out. His mother, on the other hand, wasn't having it. Because he was still a minor, the officers called her. They explained the crime to her, but when she heard the date, she cut them off. "This couldn't have been my son," she said. "How could you be so sure?" the cops pressed. "Because he was already arrested by then," she snapped back, explaining his gun arrest. The cops were dumbfounded. "Do you have a receipt or any proof?" they asked. "Yeah, I'll bring it right down," she said.

As Roy waited for his mom, he just kept his head down. He didn't want to make eye contact with the wrong cop, or the wrong man in a cell. When he did make eye contact with someone, he was grilled, heavily. He took that as a sign to just mind his business. Roy's mother arrived at the station and showed the officers the receipt, proving he was previously arrested and had been at Rikers Island at the time of this alleged robbery. These cops were determined to keep him, though, so they changed the date. "They were like, 'Nah, we gave you a mistake on the phone. It was actually on this day,'" Roy says, recalling the confusion. "Even if it happened on this day, my son was at a party with me that day," his mother said. As his mother vehemently defended him, Roy just kept watching her. She didn't seem fearful the way he was. She was determined to make sure her son wasn't arrested that day. Either the police realized they had the wrong guy, or they just realized they had come face-to-face with the wrong mother. Whatever the reason, they let him go. Six months later, Roy was arrested for armed robbery.

This wasn't the only time the police tried to put something on him that he didn't do. It made him jaded about law enforcement. He committed crimes and takes responsibility for them, but he had trouble respecting the police. "I went through prison saying if I ever got out, I'm never calling the cops for anything at all," he says. Though he doesn't feel as strongly about it today, he's still never once called the police. In his role, he can't have any real contact with the police. He'll work with the community affairs office to get permits for their events and make sure the city is aware of the routes they'll be taking when they hold marches, but outside of that "there's no real interaction," he says.

But that doesn't mean he thinks the police have no role in addressing gun violence; he knows in his heart that they do. "Their role is to get the person with the gun off the street. That's their role. They're about enforcement," Roy explains, knowing that he himself fit into that exact category when he was a teenager. "Should that kid be sent to prison for a mandatory minimum sentence, or do we put them in a program and try to redirect their behavior and redirect their thinking? Do we try to teach that kid or just lock them up?" Roy asks. "Those are different questions."

He's right: that's a different and necessary discussion. When it comes to gun violence, though, law enforcement has to be part of the solution. There is no way around that. For the foreseeable future, the police will be here. They will be part of society. People who live in these neighborhoods want the police to protect the community. They want them to hold shooters accountable. "When you think about people who are victims of gun violence, there is a piece of pain and hurt that comes with that," Roy says. "I've had conversations with parents who lose someone to gun violence and they call for justice. I can't interfere with their calls for justice. They have every right to go call for that type of justice. I think that law enforcement is there to assist with that." There are violent criminals in these communities who simply need to be off the streets. Social service workers, community leaders, violence interrupters, and other community-led workers can't arrest them and take them off the streets. The police can.

Still, their flaws are significant.

When it comes to shootings, homicides, and overall crime in disenfranchised Black communities, police struggle to have a positive, large-scale impact. Look at Roy's situation. How is it that the police were unable to figure out that they had someone who was already arrested and already had a case in the system? How could they believe Roy was involved in a robbery committed on a date that he was already locked up? Though this example is from over 30 years ago, it's an incident that could still happen nowadays.

LaTanya Gordon, the mother who lost two sons to two separate shooting incidents in Chicago in 2020, has repeatedly tried to provide the police with information about who she believes the shooter is. She's not the only one. Others in the community who know about the situation and are close to it believe this same person is the shooter. "Myself and others have given the police information pertaining to this man. Him on Facebook bragging about both murders," LaTanya declares, frustrated. After her sons were killed, a local charity donated a poster to LaTanya, a memorial of her sons. LaTanya says the shooter stole the poster and put a video of himself on Facebook pointing a gun at the poster. The caption on the video allegedly said, "I got both of these boys. The opps [enemies] got them." LaTanya spent months in 2020 providing the police with all of this information, but it never led to anything. She was told that they need a witness to come forward. All the Chicago Police Department says is that they're still investigating. LaTanya says they aren't doing enough. "They're not listening to people in the streets," she says.

Tamar Manasseh is a native of the South Side of the city. In response to gun violence in her community, she started Mothers/Men Against Senseless Killings (MASK) in 2015. It's not a typical violence prevention group. "What we started doing was setting up on a corner where we knew gun violence was most likely to occur and cooked dinner every night, seven days a week," Tamar explains. "The idea is if we're sitting on this corner and you know this is a hot spot and you know that retaliation and the cycle of violence happens in places like this, if there are mothers here, you can disrupt that cycle. Nobody wants to shoot anybody's mother and nobody wants to shoot anybody in front of someone's mother." It started with a few mothers and has now grown to a large group of people. During the summer months, the group cooks, serves food, and hangs out as a deterrence. Kids are usually around. It's a feel-good area to be in when things are calm. Tamar and the other volunteers reject the title of activist and don't view their group as an antiviolence movement. They just think it's the right thing for them to do as mothers and community members. Their presence doesn't prevent all instances of gun violence. In the summer of 2019, two MASK volunteers were killed in a drive-by shooting. Tamar hasn't let this stop the work.

She's seen law enforcement's inability to get a handle on gun crimes in her neighborhood. During the summer of 2020, a young man was shot and killed a block away from where the MASK group was set up. The killing was the result of a conflict between two opposing gangs. As with many of these murders, the community was well aware of what happened, and they knew there was going to be retaliation. There's a popular phrase that law enforcement likes to preach to community members who live in the hood where crime is prevalent: if you see something, say something. Well, that's exactly what Tamar did. There was a funeral the next week for the murdered young man. The word on the street was that something was going down at that funeral, either before or after it. Tamar told the police that they needed to be present at it. "I said you are going to need all hands on deck for this funeral," Tamar says. She didn't stop there: she also sent the police text messages, reiterating that they needed to be on alert. Based on what she heard, their presence needed to be felt at this funeral to dissuade anyone from trying something. Tamar was not the only one to warn the police.

But it all fell on deaf ears. The funeral happened on July 21 at Rhodes Funeral Services on the South Side. Dozens went to the ceremony, including family members and associates of the young man who was laid to rest. Around six thirty that evening, after the service ended, a group left the building, passing other funeralgoers who were already outside. The small group was walking down the block when a car pulled up to them. Two men got out and shot at them. Members of the walking group didn't hesitate to fire back. The shoot-out was quick, and the driver tried to leave as the ones on the sidewalk kept firing. The car crashed farther up the block, and three men bolted from it.

In total, 15 people were shot at this funeral. Even though nobody was killed, it was one of the worst mass shooting incidents on the South Side. As if that weren't bad enough, there's a police station a handful of blocks east of the funeral home. In the chaos, one person was arrested, but he was eventually released. What made it more frustrating for Tamar was that the mayor and police chief had a press conference not long after the shooting and chastised the community for not stepping up to provide information about the incident. "So if I'm seeing something and I'm saying something but you're not listening to what I'm saying, then what?" Tamar asks. That's a question many people who live in the hood have. Today, the police don't have much credibility in these communities. People don't trust them. Even law-abiding citizens who don't live by the street code distrust the police. The police don't have any real connection to the people who live in these neighborhoods.

There are also outright lawless actions by law enforcement that erode their relationship with the communities they're supposed to protect. These are not actions that are straight-up evil, like planting a weapon on an unarmed suspect the cops shot, or stealing drugs and drug money from suspects, or keeping evidence out of a case. This is about the more mundane, day-to-day misconduct that can be found in many large police departments in the country. Take the Breonna Taylor case in Louisville, Kentucky, for instance, which was one of the incidents that led to the racial reckoning in 2020. What really drew people's outrage about that tragedy was the fact that the cops shot into her apartment after serving a no-knock warrant. Because her boyfriend fired the first shot at the cops, they were within their legal right to fire back, even though neither Taylor nor her boyfriend was the target of the police investigation. So why were the cops even there in the first place? The Louisville Police Department's Place-Based Investigations Unit was investigating Taylor's ex-boyfriend Jamarcus Glover, a drug dealer whom law enforcement was trying to take down. Two detectives in the special unit, Kelly Goodlett and Joshua Jaynes, saw Glover get a package from Taylor's apartment in January 2020.

They assumed the package contained drugs but needed proof to back that up if they wanted it to be part of their overall investigation. So they tried to find evidence. Nothing came up. There was no proof that the package contained drugs and no proof that Taylor received anything in her mail for Glover on a consistent basis. The detectives weren't satisfied, so they allegedly falsified an affidavit requesting a no-knock warrant on Taylor's home. The affidavit included false corroboration from the postal inspector that said Glover got packages delivered on his behalf to Taylor. The fake affidavit led to the no-knock warrant, which led to the SWAT officers serving that warrant at Taylor's home, which led to her boyfriend firing at the officers, mistaking them for intruders, which then led to Taylor's death as a result of the officers shooting back. To make matters worse, after Taylor was killed, Goodlett and Jaynes allegedly worked together to write a false police report, trying to cover up the affidavit. It didn't work; the federal government charged them for these actions in 2022. That's a staggering series of events, and though this specific type of tragic outcome may not be too common, the actions of the detectives are unfortunately routine within police departments. It is part of police culture to tell a small lie on a warrant application, or say you surveilled someone you didn't actually surveil, or tell your supervisor you saw drugs in the car of someone you arrested when you didn't actually see any.

The Breonna Taylor killing, the funeral shooting in Chicago, the investigation into the murders of LaTanya's sons, and what happened with Roy when he was a kid at the police station—all show a lack of strategy on the part of the police. This connects to how law enforcement addresses crime, specifically gun crimes in the hood. The police aren't trusted in the hood. Without trust, it's harder to solve the killings that happen. When they can't solve the killings, perpetrators don't have much fear about shooting someone, because they know the police likely won't find them or have enough evidence to arrest them. In turn, the police aren't able to protect the communities. And of course, the unnecessary violence that police inflict on community members doesn't help either. Why would anyone trust the police if their only experience with them is being harassed and aggressively detained? Remember, it's not just about the police shooting and killing someone. Being violent with residents—not just the violent criminals but everyday citizens—in the community has dire ramifications. The police can fall into the habit of treating everyone in the hood like a criminal. That makes people believe the police aren't there to protect them but rather are there to hurt and prey on them. What's the most basic function of law enforcement? To protect and serve the taxpayers and get violent criminals off the streets. When done right, policing can prevent crime. Good police work keeps a city safe.

Law enforcement needs to be more strategic. In areas that really struggle with shootings and homicides, the police shouldn't focus on the minuscule or certain nonviolent issues. Cops aren't social workers. Instead of sending police by themselves to a call about someone having a mental health emergency, a mobile crisis unit can try to handle the situation first. Those workers possess far more training to handle such incidents. This doesn't mean police should be replaced by social workers. If the situation has the potential to get dangerous or violent, then an officer can be on standby while the trained social worker takes the lead. But the police should take a step back from the nonviolent incidents that they tend to get involved in. Cities have already rolled out these co-responder programs. We have to reduce the burden on the police. They don't have the tools or skills to do all the things certain cities ask them to do. It's unfair to community residents and unfair to the police.

The police can still patrol, but not just to harass Black citizens. There is a function to having cops patrol the streets. It helps preserve public safety around commercial areas, schools, and churches, and it makes the city and neighborhood viable. Quality-of-life policing is useful if it's done the right way; it also helps the police build a relationship with those in the community. The wrong way is something like what Philadelphia did in 2022. The city expanded its youth curfew and had police officers enforce it more stringently in the hope of addressing violent crime, even though all the available data show that curfews have no impact on violent crime and gun violence. Instead of decreasing gun violence, it just led to more teenagers being detained when they were outside late and created more animosity between the kids and the police. That's bad policing. It's not illegal, and the cops didn't do anything wrong, but did it help the youth in the city? Halfway through 2023, shootings and homicides had decreased in Philadelphia compared with the previous year, but youth homicides had risen significantly.

Community policing sometimes has a negative connotation attached to it from the perspective of criminal justice researchers, but that's usually when it's used as a sole solution. Beat cops getting to know people and developing an authentic connection is a net positive. "I love the fact that people know my name and know that they can call me at any time. I made an effort to be that type of officer. A familiar face," one St. Louis officer says. But it's pri-marily the beat and uniform cops who build such relationships with the community. The investigative teams and units are the ones who are actually going to reduce crime in a meaningful way. While focusing on violent crime, these units need to be more pro-active in their investigations but also do more retroactive investi-gations. It sounds contradictory, but it makes sense in action.

Proactive policing, or problem-oriented policing, is a critical component of all of this. For the police to be proactive, they need to identify the people who are driving the violence and the "hot spots," as they're known in criminal justice circles. As any com-munity leader or expert would explain, most of the violence in these neighborhoods is concentrated within a small set of people and locations. The police have to identify these, but how? They must gather intelligence. Building a relationship and sense of trust with community members will help them get that information, which will allow them to be more aware of where the violence is occurring and who is involved in it. They should also use data to gather this information. Shooting incident data (like the kind ShotSpotter tracks), mapping, and social media tracking would help the police have an even more comprehensive understanding of the whos, whats, wheres, and whys.

With all this information gathered and tracked on a regular ba-sis, they can work to figure out how to best combat the violence, whether that's conducting a prolonged investigation into a certain group, patrolling a specific area within the hot spot, or identify-ing someone who could be an informant for them. The police will be able to determine the proper action after putting in proactive efforts. "You have to step up your intelligence gathering. You have to get out into the neighborhoods and talk to people and figure out what's going on," Dan Isom, former commissioner of the St. Louis Police Department, says. Dan was also the director of public safety for the city of St. Louis when they had a record year of homicides in 2020, largely driven by gun violence. The next year saw a dramatic decrease, which Dan credits to a changed effort and strategy from the police. "We really changed our deployment of officers to a presence in neighborhoods at times and locations where things are likely to occur," he adds. "We made an effort to build trust and confidence in the community."

Like any other solution to this problem, it's not perfect. These types of measures can lead to the criminalization of certain people, especially if the police are focused on one specific area in a neighborhood. In Brownsville, Brooklyn, if the police know that the Tilden Houses on Dumont between Rockaway and Mother Gaston Boulevard are a hot spot, then it's possible (and historically very likely) that every single person who lives on that block will be susceptible to stigmatization, harassment, and brutality at the hands of the police. "There are positive aspects, but there are also some negative consequences in terms of placing people on a specific list. What does that do in terms of stigmatizing those individuals? How are their rights being violated?" Dr. Joseph Richardson asks. That is why problem-oriented policing must include collaboration with residents and community leaders. It needs to be fair and just.

Some actions have been taken to address unjust and abusive policing at the federal and state levels. Forty-five states have passed some type of law enforcement reform. In 2022, President Joe Biden signed an executive order to advance police accountability and help build trust in law enforcement. It hits all the points that experts call for to improve policing: limiting the use of force, banning chokeholds, using more body cameras, conducting more timely investigations into misconduct, and improving data collection and transparency. Both sides tend to roll their eyes at initiatives like this. Those on the right say they're too restricting, and people on the left say they don't do anything to address the problem. It's hard for 18,000 independent police agencies to all change at the same time. Remember, police brutality is related to gun violence because the brutality affects how well the police do their jobs. Mandated reform for police departments is a nice step, but it means nothing if the departments themselves don't truly change and adapt their strategies. All the cities that had yearslong federal investigations into their police departments still struggled significantly with crime and with the dynamic between police and the community. Plus, every department and community is different. As in addressing gun violence, there isn't a "one size fits all" solution to improving police departments. What all of them should do is focus on crime prevention and habitual violent criminals. The departments have to invest in better training along with fair and effective policing that not only reduces crime but improves community relations. The strategy has to be specific to each department and city. Criminal justice experts have pointed out how short-staffed police departments have been since the summer of 2020. If these departments improved their strategies and showed that they're there to help the community, then maybe more people would want to sign up to be cops.

William Bratton, the famed, albeit controversial, NYPD police commissioner from 1994 to 1996, was instrumental in developing the idea that law enforcement should be more proactive. He, along with others, came up with the CompStat system, which tracks crimes in New York City. Many other cities would adopt and implement this program or a very similar version of it. The program gave the NYPD the ability to track and identify hot spots, identify patterns, and, more importantly, track repeat offenders. "We had a timely, accurate system for identifying where crime was occurring, when it was occurring, and who was doing it as well as the victims," Bratton explains. The implementation of CompStat coincided with the decrease in shootings and homicides that New York City started to experience in the 1990s. "The drop came about largely from police efforts to be more proactive in going after gun crimes," the former commissioner says. But what else coincided with that drop? Mass incarceration, specifically of Black men. This wasn't all on the decision-makers. Black leaders in these communities wanted to see their cities get tougher on crime as well. Politicians and city leaders listened to those leaders and went after all the criminals they could find. That's how nonviolent drug offenders ended up in prison for years.

But at the time, no one was worried about mass incarceration; the focus was on addressing crime, and problem-oriented policing was producing too many results. Operation Ceasefire was part of that push. Developed by criminologist David Kennedy, the author of *Don't Shoot*, Ceasefire was implemented in Boston in 1996, after the city dealt with years of rising gun violence among youth. Ceasefire targeted the youth population and the hot spots that were struggling with shootings and homicides. It was a coordinated effort involving the police, the court system, gang outreach and prevention workers, clergy, and other community-oriented workers and programs. The idea of the program was to shut down the open-air drug markets and reduce shootings by dealing with those involved in a face-to-face manner. "Right before we kicked off Operation Cease Fire, we had one month in Boston in which we lost 12 kids to homicide. It was not in the power of combined Boston law enforcement to go address those 12 gangs," David previously said. "So we said something very simple. We said, 'This is about the violence. And the next gang in Boston that puts a body on the ground, we're going to go there and we're going to roll them up.'" If the community members, outreach workers, and leaders couldn't convince the youth to stop the shootings, the authorities— using proactive techniques to identify the hot spots and people consistently involved in shootings—would go after them.

David explained how they engaged with the gangs in Boston that were responsible for most of the shootings: "We had two meetings. The first meeting was to announce a gang crackdown that had already happened. It was to say, 'We did this. This is how we're operating now.' . . . We saw gangs start to act up and we sent messengers to them. This is about talking to people. And the messengers said, 'You're acting up. We're watching. Don't let it go any further because, if it does, we're going to do to you what we did to these other people.'"

While it was being used, the program was deeply analyzed from a qualitative and quantitative perspective to see what type of impact it had. The results on the ground showed that Ceasefire was associated with a sizable reduction in youth homicides in Boston, specifically in the Mattapan, Dorchester, and Roxbury areas where the program was focused. Criminal justice researchers, law enforcement, and others in the crime world praised the program. David went on to help the police department in Minneapolis implement their own version of it. Other departments across the country started integrating its principles into their policing methods. It wasn't always the exact same model, which created some issues with how people viewed the program and how effective it was. Still, it involved the kind of policing that can make an impact. Another term for this is focused deterrence, where law enforcement, social services, and other groups put all their attention on the most at-risk offenders in a community. It can look different in every place, but Ceasefire set the model.

Today, though, some law enforcement officials believe that it's become more difficult for the police to be as proactive. Part of that has to do with crime data collecting, which at the national level is downright horrendous—the federal government needs to significantly improve how it collects national crime data. But as former NYPD commissioner William Bratton says, "The problem is now getting the proper coordination and cooperation from district attorneys that are part of the criminal justice reform movement who are trying to keep as many kids out of jail as possible. It's well intended but the reality is that despite the best efforts of people, there are bad people and criminals that need to be separate from the rest of the population." It's a harsh reality for some in the reform community to accept. Nationally over 40 percent of people who are locked up were incarcerated for crimes classified as violent. It's not always clear what the term "violent crime" refers to from a legal standpoint, but it's fair to say that anyone who is locked up for a shooting or murder is a violent criminal. Plus, many of them are there as repeat offenders. But if local district attorneys' offices are not taking part in the coordinated effort for law enforcement to be more proactive in their policing, then it makes the goal of getting violent criminals off the streets more difficult to achieve. And who's to say certain violent criminals can't change in prison? After all, that's supposed to be the point of prison. Look at Roy.

There needs to be a middle ground with proactive policing. For law enforcement to address the surge in gun violence and not make the same mistake of locking up as many people as possible, they need to include the community in their proactive measures, especially through community-led initiatives that can help in the long term. District attorneys' offices have to take part in the coordination. Ceasefire is a great blueprint for them in today's climate. But you don't even have to go back that far. Remember, before 2020, the country was in the midst of a decline in shootings and homicides. That wasn't a fluke. Some real actions were being taken on the ground in many of these struggling neighborhoods. East New York in Brooklyn—where the 75th Precinct is located and where Roy was detained back in the early 1990s—had remarkable numbers in 2018. There was a stretch of over 100 days where a murder did not occur. This was credited to the efforts of the police, along with the help of community members, to go after the gangs and the guns. Violence interrupters were credited with the decrease as well. Chicago also had a decline in 2018, which was viewed in part as a result of the police working with data analysts

to track trends, predict violence, and send out the proper resources. It was a both-and approach.

Proactive policing can be effective if done properly. In 2022,
George Mason University criminologist David Weisburd did a
study with several colleagues that examined hot-spot policing
done with respect for residents. The researchers went to high-risk
areas in three cities, Houston, Tucson, and Cambridge, Massachusetts. Officers were assigned hot spots to focus on in the cities, and half of the officers received training on treating residents
fairly and respectfully. The researchers found 14 percent less
crime in the areas with officers who had received the training,
compared with the other hot spots. The officers did their jobs
better when they treated people with respect. This was after the
pandemic, the murder of George Floyd, and the social unrest.
People in these communities are more than willing to accept
the police. It would actually be more accurate to say that they
want the police present. All the police need to do is treat them
with respect and only target the ones who are committing violent
crimes. That's how they can build trust. This all connects to how
officers are trained as well, which goes back to strategy. Instead
of training officers to operate like they're in a war zone (and
arm them with military-level equipment they rarely use), train
them to be respectful and fair.

This touches on a specific aspect of the targeted policing strategy: the elite anticrime squads that departments have turned to
for decades as a response to violent crime. The teams are typically
small groups of police officers who go out into the streets to sup-
press violent crime. They use aggressive tactics to go after their
targets. Many of these officers walk around in regular clothing;
they often do not look like police to the untrained eye. Think of the
Gun Trace Task Force in Baltimore and what their mandate was.
The priority was to get guns and violent criminals off the streets
at all costs.

Many of these units became corrupt, routinely abused their power, and operated with very little oversight in the streets. There have been scandals involving elite police squads in New York City, Los Angeles, Chicago, and Atlanta. There has been a lot of debate about these units, especially after high-profile tragedies like when Tyre Nichols was beaten to death in 2023 by officers who were part of Memphis's Street Crimes Operation to Restore Peace in Our Neighborhoods (SCORPION) unit. Any honest police officer who saw the videos of Nichols's death would tell you right away that those officers were not following any standard policing practices. They looked like criminals beating up someone they had an issue with. "We witnessed a horrific crime committed by people who knew what they were doing and did not feel like they would be held accountable for it," says Ronal Serpas, a former police chief in Nashville and New Orleans who worked in law enforcement for 34 years.

People in the hood perceive that lack of accountability in all police, but especially the officers who are part of specialized teams. It's like they can walk around and do whatever they want unless they get caught on camera or kill someone who wasn't a criminal. If we're going to keep specialized anticrime units, they have to adopt a more strategic approach. It starts with leadership: these units need to have hypervigilant supervision. There needs to be a clear goal and a clear strategy from the top. The commanding officer must know what the members are doing to carry out the plan. If units like this are to be given license to move freely throughout the city in search of shooters and other violent criminals, then they need much more oversight. That goes for all police officers. There needs to be more accountability and self-policing, especially from law enforcement leaders.

At the same time, the elite units can adopt a policing method that is more focused on hot spots, just as the investigative arms of the department should. The elite teams can narrow their focus and target their enforcement on known individuals who are committing violent crimes or carrying illegal weapons. This is not the zero-tolerance strategy followed by most elite crime units, which stop everyone that moves and view everyone as a threat. That's not good policing. They need to focus on the specific people who they know are the shooters and violent criminals. And if they aren't sure, then they have to build intelligence and relationships with people in the community. "If departments are following the precepts of hot-spot policing, we know that it reduces crime. This hot-spot stuff has been around for a long time," Serpas says. There are dozens of studies on this strategy that show its effectiveness. If we're going to keep these elite units, then they need that strategy guiding them. They need to be guardians of the community.

That's the proactive side. The police also need to put their efforts into retroactive investigations of violent crime and property crimes. What does that mean? Let's revisit the city of Boston. In 1991, the city's police decided to gather the names of all the people who kept showing up in police files and reports, guys who had been caught with a gun a couple of times or had been identified by a witness in a shooting investigation only to have the witness get scared and refuse to talk: essentially the people the police knew were the players. The police made a list of about 100 of those individuals and then went after them. Did they get them for murder? Not in all cases, but they got them for other things like parole violations or carrying a gun. They made these people the priority of their investigations and build strong cases against them so they could be prosecuted by the district attorney. These suspects all got time off the streets. After that, the murder rate went down by 40 percent for two years. That's simple and fundamental policing.

Working backward and working forward around shootings and homicides, while also improving crime data collecting, is what the police should be putting their time and energy into, not menial work that just produces stats and cleared cases. So why do police struggle with this today on a grand scale? In the 1980s and '90s, it wasn't just about addressing crime. Politicians took aim at drug use and drug dealers, especially in poor Black communities. Because it was a focal point for politicians, it became a focal point for police departments, and they began placing an emphasis on drug prohibition and drug enforcement. After passage of the 1994 crime bill, the focus was on mass arrests, incarceration, and drug seizures. It was all about the war on drugs and the broken windows theory, which is the idea that if an area looks run down, then people are more likely to commit small crimes that could lead to more serious crimes. So if there's a warehouse on the block in the hood that has a bunch of broken windows, ripped fences, and front doors hanging off the hinges, then criminals will be more encouraged to commit crimes there. Law enforcement—particularly in New York—decided to focus on minor crimes like loitering, vandalism, drinking in public, and jaywalking. The theory was that focusing on these smaller crimes would discourage people from committing more serious crimes. It would also give the impression that the police were improving the quality of life. Long-term investigations like the one done in Boston in 1991 weren't rewarded. Yes, in certain pockets of the country there was good work happening, like Ceasefire or some of the policies implemented in New York City, but on a larger scale, that wasn't the case. This created a culture of ineffective policing across the country that persists today.

As the great David Simon has preached for decades, the police need to end the war on drugs.

"The drug war destroyed police work. Police are not good social workers, they're not good community relations people. The one thing police can do is take violent repeat offenders off the street," David says. "The police do one thing well: they take out the trash, and by 'the trash' I mean the people who are harming other people. It doesn't mean locking everybody up. It doesn't mean broken windows, zero-tolerance Rudy Giuliani bullshit."

But that's what the drug war did: it made the police go after people in Black communities whom they shouldn't have gone after, which exacerbated the tension between the police and the Black population that still rages on today in America. At the peak of the war on drugs, police departments saw their arrest numbers for drug crimes go up while their arrests for murders decreased. David Simon is right: police are not good at community relations, especially in the hood, but if they want to have a sustained impact on the rate of community gun violence in America, then they need to get better at it. One of the biggest issues law enforcement faces when it comes to gun violence is solving homicides. Nationally they solve less than 50 percent of them, but within the dense urban neighborhoods it can be as low as 20 percent or 10 percent. If the victim is Black and poor, it's easy to get away with murder in America. "It's no secret why we can't solve a lot of these homicides," a Chicago homicide detective says. "If people are afraid to talk to us or don't want to come forward, then we failed. We have to get people to trust us and we have to protect people." If the police had a better connection to the communities they serve, they would solve more gun homicides. They'd be better at building intelligence and maintaining informants. Detectives want to solve these cases. But they're part of a culture that has done so much damage to these communities that they don't have any trust. If people felt like the police were there to help and not to harass, arrest, and brutalize them, then they'd be more than happy to talk with them. The police and politicians need to give up on the drug war. They lost that war a long time ago. If they want to solve shooting deaths, police need a connection to the neighborhoods and those who live there.

This is especially the case in a small city like Youngstown, Ohio. Over 60 miles north of Pittsburgh, the downtown area of

Youngstown is a fraction of the size of New York City. You could describe Youngstown as a mini-Detroit. It was once a city of 170,000 people and one of the largest steel producers in the country, but now there are just over 60,000 people. The steel industry and the jobs that came along with it vanished. Aside from the large structures that are part of Youngstown State University—the football field and the stadium where the basketball team plays— some of the biggest buildings are the old mansions that mafia members used to live in when the city was a mob stronghold. Residential areas are spread out and less dense than those in a big metropolitan city. That's partly because houses have been torn down, as have many of the giant mills that used to employ people and drove the economy of the city. The homes that remain look like they could be abandoned, even the ones that people live in. The businesses do as well. A number of gas stations have been out of commission for so long that weeds grow where the pumps used to be. Youngstown is a poor city. It has all the struggles with crime and gun violence that big cities do; it just gets less attention.

The national surge in gun violence that happened was no different in Youngstown. The pandemic exposed poverty in the city. The public schools were shut down, but the private schools only closed for a short period. "The cause of the violence was an accumulation of things, and I think the cure is going to be an accumulation of things," says Guy Burney, who runs the Community Initiative to Reduce Violence (CIRV) in Youngstown and is a native of Youngstown. CIRV fits into the holistic approach to addressing gun violence that has been stressed over the past couple of years. They have prevention, intervention, and intensive intervention methods to handle crime in the city. "My whole duty is to look to how to engage the community and to give them their power to help reduce the issues that we have," Guy says. According to all the young people whom he engages with and hears from, social media was a big driving factor in the spike in violence in

Youngstown in 2020. "During COVID they didn't even see the other kids they were beefing with. It was all over social media, and once you beef back it was over with," Guy explains. "I think being isolated and being on social media helped stir and put more fire on the conflict."

The murder of George Floyd had a severe impact. Not in the sense of protesting and uprisings—there were no major protests or riots in Youngstown—but in terms of the mandates for police at the time the defund movement took off. During the height of the chaos in 2020, most police departments insisted that their beat cops only interact with people if it was absolutely necessary. This was also the case for the Youngstown Police Department, which has around 140 sworn officers. "We were told to only interact with the public when you have to because of [the virus]," Youngstown police captain Jason Simon says. "Add to that officers were a little defensive because of what happened with George Floyd." The police believe that criminals saw this as an opportunity to take advantage of the "absence of guardians in the streets," as Captain Simon calls it. "We know criminals are opportunists. They knew in that moment their odds of getting away with something increased because the cops aren't out there as much."

That said, Youngstown police officials believe they have a strong relationship with residents, which is the result of years and years of work. Knowing that people were concerned about what happened in Minneapolis, they took their role very seriously. "Working with the CIRV office, we had meetings with the community, with pastors about all of this," Youngstown police chief Carl Davis says. "It can get very uncomfortable at times for people to even talk about, but it's necessary, and those conversations happen on a regular basis." And the police welcome pushback from residents and community activists. During one of the meetings in the summer of 2020, law enforcement showed the videos of Floyd's murder and the death of Rayshard Brooks, the Atlanta man who was killed by police in a Wendy's parking lot after he took one of the officers' tasers.

At the meeting—which about 50 people attended—the police wanted to have the opportunity to explain what was done wrong or right in each situation. None of the Youngstown officers found anything right in the video of Floyd's murder. There was nothing about Derek Chauvin's actions they could defend. To them it wasn't police work, it was an abuse of power. Rayshard Brooks was a different situation, though. They played the video a few times while one of the cops analyzed and explained it to the group in attendance. The police had a hard time finding anything wrong with what the cops did in that situation. "That probably would have been my response," one of the officers said. That caught people's attention. To the residents, it was wrong. They didn't believe Brooks did anything to deserve a gunshot. A pastor felt the need to challenge the police. He was visibly upset. "Why couldn't they use a taser?" he asked the officers.

"That man was running; he was just trying to get away. He wasn't going to hurt anyone," he said. The officers countered with several points. They said the two cops tried to tase him, but he hit one of the officers and took one of their tasers. The pastor still didn't think any of that should have resulted in Brooks's death. The officers agreed but said that in those situations, the cops only have so much time to make a decision, and Brooks could have put other people in danger. The pastor wanted to hear from a different officer who was at the meeting, someone he had a relationship with, who hadn't said anything about this shooting yet. He asked the officer to be honest with him and tell him if the two cops in Atlanta handled the situation correctly. "Pastor, you know I love you and I got your back, but that was the right thing for the officer to do," he said. It seemed like the pastor still wanted to debate, but he trusted this officer and respected his perspective, so he accepted it.

This was how the Youngstown police tried to handle what was a tough moment for law enforcement in the country. They took the time to listen to the concerns that community members had, but they also reminded them that the problems going on in Minneapolis weren't happening in their city. They don't have a historical pattern of discrimination like the police department in Minneapolis does. The leaders in Youngstown know they have to be proactive to have the most positive impact on gun violence. They know the importance of building relationships to help them in their efforts to stop gun crimes and to minimize the likelihood that a tragic murder like Floyd's happens. "We had meetings with the chief and the community. The mayor and the chief meet with pastors, talking about what's going on," Guy says. The police have had community members attend training sessions so they understand what the proper use of force is and what officers are and aren't allowed to do.

The relationship is the core element in effective policing. After that, it's about instituting proactive law enforcement strategies that have a real impact. They target the areas where crime tends to happen and focus on the small groups that are in conflict with one another. They're working closely with CIRV and some of the other community-led programs in the city. The police want to make sure assault-style rifles are not easily making their way into the city. "Nine millimeters are by far the most of what we see, but we are starting to see more of the AR sporting rifles," Captain Simon says. The Youngstown Police Department is small, but they're not using that to make excuses. Their role in addressing gun violence is as important as ever.

This all sounds complicated but it's not. This isn't about rhetoric or catchy phrases. The police need to be more strategic if they want to be effective against gun violence. They know what that means, and city leaders and politicians know what that means. They've heard it for years from critics. It's not a secret. End the war on drugs. Then stop the mass arrests for nonviolent and nonharmful crimes. After that, change the instructions from the top and focus on targeting the people who are committing violent crimes. That should be the number one priority for the police. They also must build a solid relationship with community leaders and organizations. This is how they'll become better at solving homicides. Have an open line of communication with them. Listen to community stakeholders—the real ones, not the ones who shout from outside the neighborhoods but are too scared to ever set foot in them. Police need to be open and transparent with the neighborhoods about what they're doing. Have a 100 percent zero-tolerance policy for unlawful police violence. This approach is harder and takes more discipline and skill. So instead of rewarding police for making a bunch of useless arrests, politicians and the federal government should reward the ones who are doing the proactive and retroactive investigations into violent crime. The feds love investing in law enforcement, so give money to the agencies that are doing it the right way. But more money is not the real answer; it's about strategy. The investment should be in making police agencies better. This is all possible—there are many examples that show it's possible. The question is, when are the police going to make a full-scale and meaningful effort to achieve it?

5

Investment

At the peak of his time on the streets as a stickup kid, there weren't many places that Roy wouldn't rob. Some of these robberies would end without violence; other times people got shot. Even after he was wrongfully detained in October 1991, he didn't stop. "That should have been a sign for me to sit back and think about what I was doing," he says. His run on the streets wouldn't last long. Roy was just 16 years old when he got caught with a gun in late 1991. The police released him on his own recognizance—meaning he was let out while the case was pending—for the gun charge. While out on this case, he started robbing again. "That was just being someone who wasn't thinking," Roy says. In April 1992, though, the police got him again.

In his indictment, Roy was charged with around 40 counts of armed robbery. "It's funny because some of the stuff I wasn't even responsible for, but once you get arrested the cops throw it all on you," Roy explains. "But how could I claim that I'm not responsible for this robbery but I am responsible for that one?" He was sentenced to 23 years in prison. He thought he was never going to come home. "That was it right there, that was going to be the rest of my life," he says.

Roy was sent to Downstate Correctional Facility, a maximum-security prison about 70 miles north of his Bed-Stuy neighborhood. Downstate, which closed in 2022, was known as a classification center. It was a facility where new prisoners would stay for a few weeks while they waited to be assigned to a permanent location. Though he was still technically a juvenile, for some reason Roy was housed with the adults.

On his way to prison, there was a pit in Roy's stomach. When he was robbing and getting into shoot-outs, he knew he would likely end up in one of two places: in the ground or in prison. Death wasn't as frightening to him. The drive to prison was terrifying. Still, he didn't have many regrets at this time. As he says, he didn't grasp the value of life yet. To him, going to prison was almost like a rite of passage for all the guys he was on the streets with. You did your work and then you went away, either to a grave or to a cell.

He'll never forget when he first got there. An officer saw him and noticed how skinny and slight he was. "You have to get some muscle on you before you leave here," the guard firmly told him. Roy just stared at him, unsure of how to respond. "Get down and give me 20 push-ups." Roy was confused. "What?" he asked. "Get down and give me 20 push-ups," the guard repeated, with a more aggressive tone. So Roy got down and did the 20, believing he didn't have a choice. By the fifth one he started to struggle, but he finished them. The guard nodded and let Roy continue into the facility.

He may have been a tough street kid back at home, but here Roy was scared. He only ate once or twice a week. "I was stressed, depressed, or whatever," he says. It didn't help that none of the food tasted good. Another inmate noticed that he wasn't eating and stressed the importance of it. "You got to get strong, you got to get your immune system up. This place will wear you down," the elderly inmate told him. As time went on, he got a little more comfortable in this facility. He played basketball on the courts outside during recreational time. He wasn't as strong and crafty as the other inmates, but Roy would leave them frozen with his first step to the basket. He also played cards with some of the older inmates. He got comfortable and somehow a little safe at Downstate. But since this was only a temporary spot for him, that comfort was fool's gold.

After three weeks at Downstate, Roy was transferred to his permanent facility, Coxsackie Correctional Facility, around 70 miles north of Downstate. Roy felt the same on the ride up there as he had on the ride to Downstate—a pit in his stomach, palms sweaty, eyes twitching. "As soon as I got there, it was like a war inside the yard. People were stabbing each other," Roy says. "I was so surprised to see that, but I got used to it fast." Once again he had to get familiar with a new facility. The only silver lining was that this was going to be his home for a long time. He wouldn't have to up and leave in a few weeks. Roy learned that the best thing for him to do was mind his own business. At the same time, there were a handful of people from his hometown there. "I saw how many people from my neighborhood were locked up," he says. He shared stories with them about their hood and what had been going on in the years since they'd left. Even though there was some semblance of community and connectivity in the prison, Roy struggled in his first few years locked up. "I was depressed and didn't know it, I was stressed and didn't know it," he says.

His mother and his grandmother died while he was away. That was a pain he had never felt before in his life. It wasn't just that they passed; it was that he wasn't there to say goodbye to them. It was the fact that they died knowing he was locked up, not knowing if he was ever going to come home again. "That level of pain and discomfort became a catalyst for me," Roy says. "I really realized that I needed to change my life."

That change started with educating himself. He went to the library. "My mom was big on being able to read," Roy says. He was a rarity because many of his fellow inmates did not know how to read. Books couldn't completely save him, though. After all, it was a prison. Trouble was hard to avoid. While gambling one day with another inmate, Roy got into a fight. Since he was viewed as the instigator, they sent him to solitary for 50 days.

During this 50-day stretch, he could only leave his cell for one hour a day. He didn't have access to the library. Luckily, there was an inmate across from him who had been in solitary for a long time. He slid magazines and books over to Roy's cell. Of all the books he read during this stretch, it was *The Autobiography of Malcolm X* that gave him perspective. "Malcolm had you thinking on another level about how systemic things are," Roy says about the book, which is considered to be one of the essential pieces of literature from the twentieth century.

Once he was out of solitary, the education continued. He read more books. If there was any word he didn't understand, he would get a dictionary and study the word. He tried to use it more in his day-to-day. It took him a while but he ended up getting his GED in 1994, while still at Coxsackie. In 1999 he transferred to Sing Sing Prison in New York, which was a little closer to New York City and allowed his family to visit. The reputation of Sing Sing frightened Roy. At that time it had a certain level of notoriety, but Roy found the opposite when he got there. "You don't want to say that any prison is good, but in terms of being able to help a person become educated, develop, grow, transform their mind, and challenge their thinking, it's where I needed to be," he says.

He became involved with a program called the Certificate in Ministry and Human Services, where he learned about the human condition and the importance of developing a community. Through this program, he earned a certificate along with 36 college credits. Those credits were transferred over to the Mercy College prison program, which had a partnership with Sing Sing. Roy earned his bachelor's degree in 2007 and got his master's degree in 2010, all while in prison. He was released in 2015. "The more I learned, the more value I saw in myself and the value in others," he says.

His prison experiences taught him a lot. He learned about himself, and he learned extensively about his community and its struggles. When Roy went to prison, he was looking for someone else to blame for all the things that he did; when he left, he took much of the accountability for his actions. "There was definitely some introspection on my part. I was a stickup kid, an armed robber, someone who carried guns, and someone who shot people. Someone who showed a great lack of respect for fellow human beings," Roy says, owning it. But multiple things can be true. Through his education, he learned that the larger-scale systemic issues in the hood play a huge role in problems like gun violence. And what is the number one systemic issue in the hood? Poverty. It was a problem before 2020 and it was made worse during and after 2020.

If this country wants to fix community gun violence in the long term, then a good place to start is by addressing the extensive poverty in the poor minority communities, and that means financially investing in those communities. The government (at both the local and federal levels) needs to commit to improving these communities on a large scale. It needs to properly fund the schools, improve the hospitals, and fix the blocks with vacant houses, stores, and lots. It can't stop there: the entire infrastructure of these neighborhoods needs to be improved, and not at the expense of the people who live there—they should not just be gentrified so that others can move in. The housing facilities for the people who live there need to be improved. The government must make sure people have access to better grocery stores and more robust and well-run social services. The government is also capable of prioritizing and creating more job opportunities and job training programs in these neighborhoods. Teenagers in these communities need to have access to summer youth opportunities. Trade schools would be a great way to provide education and job training for people who don't typically have access to any kind of training for a job that would actually provide for them and their families. Mental health services in these areas must be more proficient in providing resources for people who struggle.

This isn't a welfare check. The efforts just described do not involve handouts or just giving people money; they are about providing the basic necessities for a community to thrive. Fewer people would turn to a gun if they had access to a decent job. If you care about something, you invest in it. It's not an accident that these are the communities that have to ask for resources. From a historical perspective, the poverty and inequalities were all intentional. Today the people in these neighborhoods are not asking for anything more than to be able to live. City leaders and the federal government need to make this a top priority for addressing gun violence.

But this is a long-term effort and needs to be implemented over time. Even if every city started on the path of investment right now, it would take years for it to truly show results. "It's essential as a medium- and long-term strategy to ensure that overall levels of gun violence subside in those communities," Professor Rick Rosenfeld says. "It's not a short-run strategy. Reinvestment at a scale that's going to be noticeable and pay off is going to take time." Gun violence remains a pressing issue right now, so how can investing help at this moment? Another lesson Roy grasped while he was incarcerated was the need for more community-based solutions to the problems, which fit into the investment strategy. The proper and calculated implementation of certain community violence intervention (CVI) programs like the one for which Roy works is critical. This includes programs that use violence interrupters and credible messengers, but it also involves youth-focused programs, community-led educational programs, and local churches that do outreach in the neighborhood. They're not limited to just violence interruption. In most of these inner-city neighborhoods, all the community-led organizations also do some type of violence reduction work. Like everything else in the hood, they need more funding.

Picture a small group of Black men, three to four, who rent out a tiny space in their neighborhood. They have one 400-square-foot office on a corner in a rough part of the community. But in this tiny space, they teach young boys about how to resolve conflicts without turning to a gun or fighting. They teach these kids how to engage with one another, how to have disagreements without getting physical, and how not to feel disrespected by a rude comment. Every day, they work with anywhere from 8 to 12 kids. Now imagine if that small group of men had an entire building in their community to operate in. Instead of one little office, they could have multiple offices. Rather than 3 or 4 men, they would employ a staff of 15 to 20. What these hypothetical men are doing is a form of violence prevention, and if they had proper funding, their impact could be even greater.

These kinds of grassroots organizations are a safe haven for the communities in which they operate, and the majority of the people who do the work are not doing it for any reason other than that they care. They want to see their communities improved. They don't care about glory or praise. They just want people to be safe and have an opportunity to live their lives peacefully. That being said, CVI is probably the most popular form of violence prevention, and it's the one that a lot of cities and communities are focused on, believing they can make an immediate change. "They have a lot of impact. The connection that they have to the people can't be matched," Cheryl Riviere, the director of a violence intervention program in Baltimore, says.

Violence interruption work goes back decades. Though not the only example, Cure Violence is perhaps the most familiar violence intervention program in the country. It was founded in 2000 by Dr. Gary Slutkin, an epidemiologist who is often credited as one of the first to come up with this method during the 1990s. Some believe that it was formulated much earlier, however. "Violence intervention has been happening for a long time in disinvested, discriminated against, and excluded communities. Long before Cure Violence existed. It's been around forever. The idea of community taking care of community is not new," says Dr. Shani Buggs, who points to the Black Panthers as a group that was doing this work during their height.

Regardless of who started it, Cure Violence is the name that rings out. Many cities have implemented the program or adopted it in their own way, which means they've hired violence interrupters or credible messengers to go out into struggling communities and stop the spread of gun violence. These are people like Roy who have a high level of credibility because of their previous involvement with the streets. CVI workers are not the police, however. They don't have arresting or prosecuting power. "We have to look at the violence interrupter sector nationally the same way we look at EMTs. If we do not think that they have the ability to save lives in a way that EMTs do then we are mistaken and we are foolish," Erica Atwood says. Erica is the senior director of Philadelphia's Office of Policy and Strategic Initiatives for Criminal Justice and Public Safety and oversees the Philadelphia Violence Prevention office.

There are some promising data on the impact of Cure Violence from a variety of cities across the country. Over the past decade, independent studies of the program in Philadelphia, Chicago, New York City, Kansas City, New Orleans, and Baltimore have found some significant reductions in shootings, killings, and other violent crimes. These reductions can go as high as 56 percent in some areas. It's crucial to note that the numbers aren't citywide—they're in the catchment areas that the workers operate in, which is usually a 10-by-10 block area—but they would suggest a strong impact on the areas where the program is in place.

Aside from Cure Violence, New York City also has the Crisis Management System (CMS), which started in 2010. It's part of the mayor's office and also uses credible messengers who go out and mediate conflicts in the streets, dealing with high-risk people. The program is used in 21 precincts across New York City. From the first year until 2019, there was a 40 percent reduction in shootings across all CMS areas. There was a 30 percent reduction in areas that did not have the CMS program during that same 10-year period. Erica Ford, a renowned gun violence prevention leader in New York City, was one of the designers of CMS. She also leads an antiviolence group called Life Camp. Erica is one of the strongest voices among Black women on gun violence not just in New York City but in the country. She's well connected and has put decades into addressing this problem. "We are beyond first responders, we're on the front line. We're going before the situation happens and negotiating and mediating and interrupting," Erica says, passionately. "We're not showing up afterward. We're interrupting people in the middle of the situation, in the middle of the fight, in the middle of two people wanting guns drawn on each other."

Rapid Employment and Development Initiative Chicago (READI Chicago) is another popular CVI program. Launched in 2017, it recognizes the residents who are at the highest risk of gun violence in their catchment areas and connects them with job opportunities, supportive services, and counseling. The goal is to keep them from retreating back into the environments that contributed to their being involved in gun violence. On average, the people the program works with have been arrested 18 times, and around 75 percent of them have been the victim of a violent crime. These are people who are deeply entrenched in violence. It's hard for them to be reached by regular social services or any kind of city-led agency. Of course, READI Chicago would not be able to do this without using credible messengers. It has been reported that since 2019, in the four neighborhoods it operates in, these messengers have connected with more than 500 people, with more than 380 of them gainfully employed.

Though Cure Violence, CMS, and READI Chicago are some of the most notable examples, CVI work exists in many different forms across the country. With the renewed focus on gun violence that came in 2020, this type of work got a lot of attention. Significant criticism has been aimed its way by the criminal justice expert community, with some saying that it isn't as effective as its proponents claim, and others saying that CVI workers are getting too much glory and praise for the role they play. The critics aren't completely wrong in these assessments. In 2019, St. Louis invested $7 million to fund the implementation of Cure Violence and the program was launched in 2020. Professor Rosenfeld, who is based in St. Louis, wanted to see what kind of impact it had on the city. It's already been established what 2020 meant for gun violence in the country, and St. Louis was no exception. They recorded their highest murder rate in 50 years. In 2021, though, shooting and homicide numbers went down dramatically, which would suggest that Cure Violence was partially effective. But Professor Rosenfeld performed an analysis of Cure Violence for that year and saw that it didn't have much of an impact, at least in the first year.

"If Cure Violence reduced homicides and gun assaults and contributed to the overall reductions in these offenses between 2020 and 2021," Professor Rosenfeld previously said about the study, "we should observe greater reductions in the Cure Violence neighborhoods than in the comparison neighborhoods." According to his review, gun crimes and homicides did not go down in the neighborhoods where Cure Violence was operating any more than they did in neighborhoods that did not have the program, though Rosenfeld stresses that this is not an indictment of the program.

There are plenty of other studies that encourage a mixed response to violence interrupters among experts. John Jay College, one of the premier criminal justice schools in the country, performed an analysis of this outreach work in 2020 and found the results "promising but mixed." A 2015 study of the program in Pittsburgh that ran from 2004 to 2012 did not find any significant reductions in homicides. This study actually found that the program might have been tied to an increase in aggravated assaults and guns on the north side of the city. Even with the positive reviews in areas of Baltimore and Chicago, there are mixed reviews of it in certain other areas of those cities as well. A 2022 study of READI Chicago showed that there was a significant reduction in serious forms of violence in the areas the program operated in, as well as a reduction in arrests and people victimized, but critics still said it was too costly a venture.

So what does all of this mean? To critics, it means the program should not be significantly invested in. To supporters, it means the critical analysis of the programs with mixed results isn't objective or the program wasn't implemented properly. Critics like to say that the positive feedback from any CVI program analysis is flawed. It's all murky and there's a lot of back-and-forth. The middle ground in all of this is deep and targeted research. People have a narrow view of investment: they think it just means money. But it also means probing and evaluating. Some criminologists believe that these programs can be effective but need to be properly analyzed and assessed before they are implemented. There needs to be exhaustive research before the program is enacted in a certain neighborhood or community and while the program is being used. READI Chicago's goal is to target the most dangerous people in Chicago, people who are completely removed from everyday society. The data show that they've been pretty successful in that. Their goal is not to fix all crime in Chicago. People look at these programs and believe they're supposed to fix every issue. READI

Chicago has been mostly successful because they've been delib-erate. "It's got to be coordinated, it's got to be calculated, there's gonna be an assessment that's done," Paul Carrillo says. "It's got to be comprehensive because the issues are so complex in these communities."

It also must involve the community itself. It can't just be some outside research group, think tank, or philanthropic organization with a lot of money that parachutes into a neighborhood, has a couple of meetings with community leaders and residents, and then starts a program. Community activists across the country feel like some of these intervention programs do not allow enough say from residents and leaders who live in the neighborhoods be-ing served. So that's where a lot of these flaws and mixed reviews come from. In certain areas, the program was properly assessed before being put in place; in others it wasn't. Every community is different. Just because a violence interruption program worked a certain way in one neighborhood doesn't mean it'll work that same way somewhere else that struggles with gun violence. The effective response to gun crimes in Oakland isn't going to look entirely similar to the effective efforts in Boston. It needs to be specific to the area. A proper, comprehensive analysis includes determining who in the community should have a say and who shouldn't. Again, investment does not just mean money. "There has . . . been nowhere near the amount of investment in the field that's needed," Carrillo stresses. "It's like we're criticizing a kid for getting bad grades but we've never sat and helped the kid with their homework. We never got them a tutor. We've never given them the tools to make sure they're successful."

That's a crucial point, maybe the most important point as it re-lates to intervention programs. For all the concerns out there about these programs and whether they're effective, there hasn't been nearly enough deep analysis of them. Dr. Richardson ex-plains it clearly: "A lot of the studies that have been done have been quantitative. They're evaluating metrics." For example, a study will look at if the number of shootings went down in an area when there was some type of intervention program compared with a nearby neighborhood that did not have the program. It will also compare the number of shootings before the intervention was implemented with the number now. The studies aren't qualitative. They're not looking at why the shootings went down. They're not looking at what exactly the CVI workers are doing and how they're engaging with the at-risk people. What are their strategies for engaging with someone who is ready to shoot another person? What did the person who was going to do the shooting think about the intervention? What was their reaction to it? This is all important information that needs to be gathered to fully understand whether a specific program is working. "We still have a significant amount of work to do in terms of evaluating the programs, particularly the qualitative component. The studies don't get granular in terms of qualitative data," Dr. Richardson says.

There are certain criminal justice experts and researchers who study gun violence from a bird's-eye view and like to speak for people who live in these neighborhoods, even though they've never set foot in them or spoken to anyone who's from there. Many of these experts are white middle-aged academics who may or may not have been in law enforcement. If they have been, chances are it was for a quick minute before they realized how dangerous the profession is. Either way, that group has become very skeptical of all community and social programs. To them, policing is the only answer, even though there are encouraging data that show that certain intervention strategies outside of law enforcement can have a significant and lasting impact. They look at the problem as an either-or situation: either we use law enforcement, or we use community social programs.

It turns out people in the hood are a bit savvier than these academics and researchers. If you actually speak with people in these communities, you'll find they support the idea of violence interrupters and CVI. They want more community-led efforts to address gun violence, and they want to try everything that can be tried. They support both policing and community-led programs. To those who say violence intervention isn't effective, Erica asks, "Tell me, what is? Based on the same analysis you're making of this, tell us what works perfectly." The overall results of CVI aren't 100 percent glowing, which can be said about every method the country uses to address crime (the police don't only produce wins either). That doesn't mean violence interruption or the police should be abandoned; it means they need to be applied more tactically. Even the data about these programs and their results need to be more deeply explored. And guess what? People in the hood feel that way too. They're not as stupid as some of the bird's-eye experts believe they are.

There are going to be struggles and hurdles with these programs, like in Philadelphia, a city that's dealt with record shootings and homicide numbers since 2020. The city launched the Community Crisis Intervention Program (CCIP) in 2017, a violence intervention program run by a community-led organization with funding from the city's violence prevention office. In 2021 the city invested $5.3 million in the program. But an independent analysis of the CCIP in 2022 showed that it was struggling in a big way. There was a bevy of issues: understaffing, a lack of training for the workers, and a lack of leadership since there was no full-time director. It was a bad look for the city, the organization, and the community. This wasn't just a mixed review about its effectiveness: the study revealed real systemic issues with the organization. People were rightfully frustrated. They wanted answers and they wanted the program to be held accountable. It was funded with taxpayers' dollars, and taxpayers wanted answers. Did the city just abandon it? No, they decided to address the issues. The report, which was done by an independent research group, included a detailed list of recommendations for the program, which the city got to work on. We need to study the failures like that of the CCIP in Philadelphia in order to understand what works and what doesn't.

What happened in Philadelphia is not unique to that city. There are other examples of these programs having serious problems. Workers in many of the CVI programs that are struggling think the solution is more money from the government. "Everybody wants a grant, everybody wants a salary," one Brooklyn resident says, referring to certain violence intervention programs. "I'm not trying to downplay anybody's work, but I think some of these people want to be the hero of the violence." In reality, they need to demonstrate that they can be effective before they get more money. They need to prove that they can use public dollars effectively. They need to institute significant change, which is what Philadelphia vowed to do when the report came out. The point is no one is saying to throw money at these CVI programs and trust them blindly. They need to be rooted in evidence-based approaches, and those approaches need to be thoroughly analyzed and evaluated. If they want government funds, they need to be open to some type of oversight and some type of controlled trial to make sure they actually work. There has to be some vetting and accountability. Just because someone has lived experience around gun violence doesn't mean they're suited to be a CVI worker. On the public side, people need to be more patient and give these programs a chance to succeed. But critics don't even want to do that. All that being said, intervention is just one side of it. There's more investment to be done. Detractors who disparage the calls for investment think it's all about CVI. But it's about these communities as a whole and what they look and feel like.

Pastor Donovan Price is part of the community in Chicago, a city that gets targeted by everyone as a prime example of what gun violence looks like in the country and what impact it has on certain communities when it goes unchecked. It's not the entire city of Chicago that's plagued by this. It's mostly the South Side, where the notorious Parkway Garden Homes, commonly known as O Block, is located. It's a gated complex with about 35 buildings. Some of the housing projects are set up almost like triangles if you look at them from the sky. On the east side of the complex, you'll find multiple shops, including a supermarket that has a painted mural of King Von, a popular rapper from O Block who was shot and killed in Atlanta in 2020. On that same east side is an elevated train station, surrounded by inner-city strongholds. Under the tracks are more stores and shops. Apartment buildings and houses are all over. The exteriors of these homes are nice. They look as if they were built a while ago. Some are in good condition, others not so much. It's a similar layout to New York City, but the streets are wider, with more space for cars. Entire areas appear neglected, like the corner of Dr. Martin Luther King Drive and East 61st Street, where a food store, medical center, and another food market are present but all look dilapidated. Under the same train station is a very detailed piece of artwork painted on a building, right off South Vernon Avenue. It reads, "Chicago respect our city kids. Stop the violence."

Progressive Missionary Baptist Church, the church Pastor Price and four other pastors work at, is less than five miles away from O Block. Price is in his late 50s, has lived in Chicago most of his life, and started studying to be a pastor when he was 7. But he's not just an everyday church leader—he provides a particular service for the relatives of gun violence victims. "When a person is shot and killed in Chicago, in particular those that are declared dead at the scene, I try to arrive around 20 minutes after shots fired and provide ministry and care for the family, friends, witnesses, and community," Pastor Price says. "After the crime scene, I transport or accompany the immediate family to the medical examiner's office for body identification, conduct a candlelight vigil, and play an integral part in the funeral and memorial service. I also attempt to point the family in the direction of resources that can help them heal long term."

Each day, he drives around the city to do his work. It's impossible for him to respond to every single shooting, but he gets to dozens and dozens of incidents a day. "I try to be at 30 percent of all the shooting homicides in the city each year," he says. All of this started for him in 2016 when Chicago had one of its worst years of shootings and killings. It seems like the city has always been the showpiece for gun violence in America, but all of this awareness really started in 2015 after the horrific murder of 9-year-old Tyshawn Lee. Tyshawn was lured into an alley by several gang members—who were rivals of the boy's father—and shot in a retaliation execution. Pastor Price knew Tyshawn and his family. "He walked by my church all the time, dribbling his little basketball," the pastor says. This shooting drew everyone's attention to the carnage in Chicago and partly inspired Pastor Price to start doing victim outreach work. It hasn't been an easy road. He's seen entire families lose their lives to gun violence. One of the first victims he helped was a 6-year-old girl who was shot but survived back in 2016. Two years later, though, her uncle was killed. A few years after that, her mother and brother were shot and killed. He remembers an awful case where a young kid he described as a "nerd" got into an argument with some other kids on Facebook. "He was talking all that gang lingo," Pastor Price says. The next day, he ran into some real gang members and they shot him in the head. "A 20-minute virtual fight turned into a kid losing his life. A good kid," he says.

More cooperation from the city would be helpful. The Chicago Police Department has an information tool known as the Crime Prevention and Information Center, which alerts city agencies and some community organizations about crimes and provides details about them. The pastor has been trying to get access to it for years, but he's been "getting the runaround." He says there are those in the city who chirp behind his back and criticize what he does. "A lot of people give me heat about all the praying they see me do with the families," he says. "I believe in the power of prayer. I do this to provide a service and out of love with really no regard for myself or money," he explains. The talking behind his back is discouraging, but it would never stop him. "Imagine what would be happening if nobody was praying for our communities," he says.

The summer of 2020 was bad in Chicago. Pastor Price says that was the busiest time he ever had responding to shootings. The nights were deadly: he would finish up at one incident, get in his car, turn on his police scanner, and immediately hear about another shooting a few blocks away. "It was everything—the gangs were going at each other, more people had guns. It was crazy," he recalls. One particular incident he responded to was on the night of July 4, 2020. Even with all that was going on that summer, people still made time to be with their friends and family to celebrate the holiday. This is what the Wallace family did in the South Austin neighborhood that night. Natalia Wallace, a 7-year-old, was playing with some other kids outside her grandmother's house. The adults were outside too, enjoying the party.

Then it all changed when a car drove up to the house. Several people got out, took out guns, and started firing. Of course, Natalia wasn't the target—it was another person at the party, a man who was wounded in the shooting—but she was the one who got killed. Her entire family was with her when she got shot. "She left out the house, two minutes. I came out here and my grandbaby was laying down the ground down there," her grandmother, Linda Rogers Fulton, said at the time. "I didn't know what to do. It hurt me. I couldn't do nothing. My baby was laying on the ground! Jesus! Help us Father!" Pastor Price responded to that shooting. His memory of it is a blur, though, similar to every other incident he's responded to in which an innocent kid was the victim. "Trying to comfort grieving mothers who just held their baby child in their final moments. It breaks my heart," he says. That was one of 53 shootings he responded to that night. Yes, 53 shootings in one night. Pastor Price's relationship with the family doesn't end after the initial contact. He tries to stay in touch with them for as long as they need. "They can call me five years later and say we need a gallon of milk. And I'm going to find it," he says.

What's most impressive about all his work is not the hours, energy, and ability to withstand trauma that it requires. It's the fact that he does this with no real financial support. One philanthropic group provides some funding and he collects donations every now and then, but his efforts are primarily funded out of his pocket. The pastor has no complaints, though—for him it's a calling. It's his role in the cycle of gun violence that afflicts the city. "We've gotten to the point of what I call the common cold situation," Pastor Price says. "There's not going to be a cure for this, but just like for the common cold, if you're treating some of the symptoms it can give you a certain level of comfort." Using that analogy, his work can be viewed as a treatment. He arrives after the incident, but caring and providing comfort for a family who has lost a loved one to a shooting is just as important as preventive measures. Imagine if Pastor Price had city funding and could employ other pastors to do this work as well and create a network of pastors who use their free time to respond to shooting incidents and provide support for the family and friends. They could probably blanket the entire city. As a healer, the pastor has probably prevented family members from retaliating. What could an entire team of people like him do? People like Pastor Price don't have the backing of their city leaders or government agencies. The decision-makers are not thinking outside the box and seeing how someone like Pastor Price is not just useful but a necessity. "The city could help, and it wouldn't cost them much, but I don't think they see the value," he says.

Just investing in antiviolence programs isn't enough. What happens after you interrupt the violence? What structures are in place to keep people from resorting to avenues that lead to violence? What resources are there for people who are victims or relatives of victims? To deal in the long term with the unrelenting violence caused by guns, cities must make a sweeping investment in these communities. "When you go anyplace where wealthy white people live, these communities fund the things that give life to people. They fund education, they fund housing, they fund the community as a whole," Erica Ford says. Social services, schools, hospitals, youth programs, and other public services in communities affected by violence were already operating at a disadvantage before 2020, and, as expected, their situation worsened afterward. "I think with more funding then there is an opportunity to do more. People would be able to set up these community-based organizations and hire staff and could bring on more programming," Roy says. "I'm from the streets. You can't isolate poverty from gun violence." This includes something like the court and justice system, which across the board has been severely underfunded. You can have the most well-funded police department in the history of your city, but if the court system can't process someone who was arrested for shooting up a block party because it's been overburdened, then the police are pretty inconsequential. The court system needs more resources too. The same goes for data collecting and research. There need to be improvements in the data-collecting process for gun deaths and injuries. If the federal government invested in an oversight program that tracks gun deaths and shooting injuries, researchers could better understand the problem.

That's why community leaders and criminal justice experts are deliberate when they say the investment has to be comprehensive. "There's so many pieces of evidence that when you make living conditions better, there's less violence," Professor Daniel Webster, from Johns Hopkins University, declares. "You have a more secure safety net, you have better schools, better infrastructure. So we have to address those things." That being said, the professor cautions that there needs to be a sense of urgency on what can and should be done right now. As he puts it, there's a little bit of a "chicken and egg" scenario because it's hard to get public and private investment in areas where people are getting shot regularly. "So it's not just that disinvestment leads to violent crime, but violent crime leads to disinvestment as well. It's a cycle," the professor explains. This is why something like CVI combined with effective law enforcement is important to lower violence more immediately so that the community can become more stable, which should lead to more investment. "When we talk about gun violence in communities that are disenfranchised, we have to look at the disparities that are pushing people to live in poverty and as a result pushes them into having a life where violent behavior becomes an option," Rashad Singletary, a leader for gun violence prevention at the mayor's office in Baltimore, says. Rashad, like others who are well versed in this issue, knows you can't point to one thing as the cause of gun violence, but he challenges people to question what the core of it is. "I would say the seed of what we're seeing has been going on for years. It's the social-economic disenfranchisement of Black and brown communities. This isn't something new," he says.

The big question is, Where is all this money supposed to come from, which adds up to billions and billions of dollars? There are several options. First, the federal government needs to step in. Instead of politicians using the issue to make their colleagues across the aisle look incompetent, they need to actually come together to make sure funds get where they need to go. If the priority is to address the socioeconomic factors that drive gun violence in order to disrupt the daily, nonstop shootings, then the federal government will need to stop avoiding the real issues and put funds into the most disenfranchised cities and communities within those cities. "Most cities are going to require federal support," Professor Rosenfeld states.

Over the past few years, some steps have been taken at the federal level to address this. In 2021, President Joe Biden proposed the Build Back Better Act, which was introduced to Congress. The bill was, in essence, going to rebuild the middle class in America after it had been slowly chipped away at for well over a decade. This bill included many provisions, most notably a $5 billion investment in evidence-based CVI programs over an eight-year period. "Community violence interventions are proven strategies for reducing gun violence in urban communities through tools other than incarceration. Because cities across the country are experiencing a historic spike in homicides, the Biden-Harris Administration is taking a number of steps to prioritize investment in community violence interventions," a statement from the White House said regarding the funds. An investment of $5 billion is nothing to ignore and certainly signals that the federal government took the issue seriously. And while the bill specifically addressed community violence prevention work, it was also supposed to make cities and communities healthier by providing them with more resources. Unfortunately, this bill was roadblocked in the Senate after passing through the House of Representatives in November 2021; the full version never passed, and a watered-down version of the bill went into law in 2022. There was still a substantial investment for CVI work included in the version that was passed.

Politicians on the right and left also found a way to work together on the Bipartisan Safer Communities Act, which was put together shortly after the Uvalde mass shooting in 2022 and quickly signed into law that summer. Though it may not have captured the mainstream attention it should have, as Connecticut senator Chris Murphy stated, the bill was "the most significant piece of anti-gun violence legislation in nearly 30 years." Senator Murphy was one of the leaders of the bill. It's more focused on addressing easy access to weapons, but there are aspects of it that target investment. It provides $250 million in funding for community-based violence prevention initiatives. There's also an emphasis on investment in mental health services for families and providing millions for school safety. It's a step in the right direction on all fronts.

In addition to passing bills, Biden's administration also has made federal funds available to cities through grant programs that are supposed to be for communities struggling with a wide array of issues like drugs, housing, infrastructure, education, and food. These are all issues that correlate with the circumstances that drive gun violence. The grants in question are available for cities to go out and get, and the leaders in struggling cities need to take advantage of them.

Even without such grants, local governments can prioritize investments in their city budgets. If you want to understand what a city thinks is important, just look at its budget. Local politicians have spent the last couple of years condemning gun violence, begging their communities to put a stop to it and take some accountability, but they have the power to do that as well. The mayor, city council, and budget office can all work together to be more deliberate in how they allocate their funds if they really want to address gun violence. Several studies show that cleaning and repairing dilapidated houses and other structures in poor neighborhoods can help decrease gun crimes. That's something city leaders should prioritize in their budget. After the economic downturn in 2020, dozens of cities launched pilot guaranteed-income programs for working-class poor people. Recipients were selected from among qualified residents by a lottery system and received anywhere from $200 to $1,000 a month. This is something more city leaders could look into, even if it's for a temporary period to allow certain families to get a little bit of a safety net. The bottom line is there's money available to address the systemic and socioeconomic issues that drive gun violence; it's just a matter of whether the government is going to prioritize those issues or continue to let them destroy communities. It has the power, so it needs to use it.

Investment is key. Not just investment in violence intervention, or education, or housing, or infrastructure, or the courts, or community programs, or social services, or mental health programs: investment across the board is critical. It has to be widespread across different avenues. More crucially, the efforts on the ground must be evidence based. This includes both community-led programs and government ones. Those are going to yield more immediate results. But beyond resources, there needs to be coordination. The CVI programs need to coordinate with the hospital violence intervention programs. Resources are great, but without coordination they're pointless. The stakeholders and leaders in these neighborhoods have to be part of the investment focus. There needs to be accountable for these programs that are using government funds. Though it's needed everywhere, it's important to note that there's a distinction between what investment looks like in a big city and what it looks like in a smaller city, especially when it comes to violence prevention. Targeted and well-thought-out investment in CVI in a city like Chicago is not going to look the same as it would in Kansas City. Until the overall infrastructures in these neighborhoods are healthy enough to meet people's basic needs, any positive actions won't be sustained.

6

Clog the Iron Pipeline

Pow. That is the sound Roy remembers hearing the first time he shot a gun. It was a thrill and a level of excitement he had never felt before. After he fired the shot up in the air outside his housing project in Brooklyn at two o'clock in the morning, he ran back inside. He stared up at the ceiling and thought, "Wow, I shot a gun." He had only seen guns before; he had never held or fired one. He felt powerful. He felt like a man, or what his definition of a man was. The men on the streets whom he respected and looked up to carried guns. He knows they shot people. It was something that stuck with him for the rest of his time out on the streets. He can remember going to basketball practice for a rec league he played in and having the gun in his waistband while he ran up and down the court. In fact, during one practice, Roy got into it with the coach. Annoyed, the coach made him run laps, but Roy didn't put enough effort into it, so the coach told him to do push-ups. As he went down on each push-up, he could feel the gun hit the gym floor.

Now all that came next was for him to shoot someone. In the late 1980s, Roy was in the courtyard of his project complex. He and a couple of friends were playing skelly, a well-known outdoor game played in the streets of New York City. The game is simple: a smooth part of the sidewalk is used as the board, where numbers are drawn within a box, usually with chalk. The number 13 is in the middle, while the numbers 1 through 12 are around the 13 in the square. Each number is within its own box. Taking turns, players try to flick a bottle cap to the 1 and then all the way to the 13. After that, they go from 13 back to 1. This game was a staple of the old New York City and Roy played it constantly during the summer months.

One of Roy's other friends arrived and explained that there was an issue with another guy in the neighborhood. He can't recall exactly what the issue was, but one of his friends suggested that Roy be the one to deal with it. "We need somebody that's gonna go out there and really show this guy what's good," Roy remembers his friend saying.

With no hesitation, Roy was in. "Let me go upstairs to get a jacket," he told his friends. What did he need a jacket for? It was August. He needed it to hide the gun. When he went up to get his jacket, the adrenaline rushed through him. He was about to go prove himself. The group of friends—around five of them—got in a car. Roy put the gun in the inside pocket of his jacket. His friends had the whole situation mapped out. They were going to drive to the block and point out the man they wanted Roy to shoot. Once they spotted him, they'd drive around the corner and let Roy and a couple of his friends out, and then Roy would do the rest. On his way to the scene, that adrenaline turned to anxiety. He was in the coat, dripping sweat. The guys in the car joked around—this was light work to them. It was not a big deal for them to be on this ride, but it was for Roy. He stared out the window as they drove, trying to lock in. He was not thinking about the value of life. He was just worried about his rep. He wanted his friends to see that he was for real. That they could trust him. That he was not afraid to do what was necessary.

When they got to the block, the guy wasn't there. Still, the driver drove around the corner and let Roy and his friend out. On the streets, it looked like any other summer day in Brooklyn. Because this was his friend's block, some of his family was out there. The friend talked and laughed with them. Roy just stood there. He usually cracked more jokes when with his friends, but that was not where he was at mentally in this moment. He was on edge. But some time went by and the guy didn't show up. Maybe he wasn't around anymore. Maybe he went to the store. Maybe he knew trouble was coming and stepped away from the block. Whatever the case, he was nowhere to be seen. It seemed like Roy might not have to carry this out. He could go back to his block and return to the skelly game.

"Oh, there he go!" Roy's friends said with excitement, pointing across the street.

It wasn't up in the air anymore. This was about to go down. They approached him with haste. The guy, a street-savvy man, knew what was up but stood his ground. He and Roy's friend started arguing. "What's all that shit you was saying?" the friend asked. The two of them went at it with words. Roy stood off to the side, just watching. The argument grew more intense until the friend was done with it. He turned to Roy. "You know what? Shoot him."

For a split second, Roy froze. The statement—which was more of a command—was no surprise. This was exactly what he was here for, but he still needed a second for it to sink in. The guy didn't wait to see what would happen. He took off. Roy pulled the gun out and fired. Everyone nearby took off. Any innocence Roy had was gone. He went from playing skelly to shooting someone without any questions asked.

"It was like seeing people run onto a football field or seeing people dispersing from a dangerous situation," Roy says, with some level of shock that he actually did it. Roy and his friend didn't wait to see if he hit the guy—they ran too, up the block to the car that drove them there, where the driver waited. He busted a U-turn and drove toward where Roy did the shooting. They wanted to see if the guy was hit. He was. Roy hit him multiple times. That satisfied Roy and his friends so they drove away, back to his apartment complex. "I was like, damn, what the hell did I just do," Roy says. But those thoughts quickly went away, because he got nothing but praise on his block. "Yo, he got a lot of heart," was something Roy was told after the fact. There's the validation he was looking for. A simple statement of admiration.

At the time, getting that admiration meant a lot to him, but what stands out to Roy now, decades later, is how easy it was for him to get his hands on a gun, as well as the fact that he and his friends didn't really understand how much power a gun carried. Just as shooting someone wasn't that big a deal, walking around with that kind of weapon wasn't a big deal. Today, as a violence prevention worker, Roy grapples a lot with what drives people to pick up a weapon. He thinks a lot about what drove him to do so. As far as he's concerned, the accessibility can't be ignored.

"It's easier to get a gun than it is for Black people in our communities to get a job," Roy declares. When he was a teenager, he had no problem getting his hands on a firearm. If he couldn't get one from his friends, there was an old-timer who would sell them to teenagers in the neighborhood. He was stealing them from docks in Brooklyn. Whatever the pipelines are for the guns to make their way into the community, Roy believes they're just as strong today as they were when he was coming up. The complaint he always hears from those in the community is that there are too many guns, which makes Roy wonder if people believe that there should be a certain number of guns but not "too many." "Do we need any guns in these communities?" Roy asks.

That's a deep question because it goes beyond any one community and touches on the rights of citizens: their right to protect and arm themselves, and the decades of work gun manufacturers and their lobbyists have done to undermine gun regulations. This is why the gun-laws aspect of firearm violence is such a sticking point for people—even though there's no way stronger gun laws won't be part of the long-term solution for addressing inner-city gun violence. Any lawmaker or city leader who suggests strengthening gun laws as a way to deal with gun violence is automatically viewed by a certain section of the population as a threat to their Second Amendment rights. Not to mention they're also routinely lobbied against by the gun industry and the National Rifle Association (NRA). That's a real component of this as well, but the discussion of gun laws rarely touches on the impact these laws have on poor Black communities. It's usually about whether law-abiding citizens have the right to own a gun and what type of gun they should be allowed to have.

America loves guns. That's why more than half of the states have permitless carry laws, which allow people to carry guns in public without needing a license. When it's easy to obtain a gun, someone is more likely to use it in situations where it's not necessary. Like when a neighbor asks a man to stop shooting his AR-15 outside their home because they have a baby sleeping, so the man goes into the neighbor's house and kills five people. Or when a senior citizen shoots a neighbor because his leaf blower is too loud. When guns are easy to obtain, day-to-day conflicts can become deadly.

Those in the gun industry, though, just want to be able to sell as many firearms as they can and not have any responsibility for what happens after that. The sad truth is the national discourse on regulating guns usually emerges after a tragic mass shooting, especially at a location where it's not "supposed" to happen. When a 12-year-old boy is shot in a car in Brooklyn, or a youth football coach is shot and killed in front of his son in Lancaster, Texas, or a barbecue in Chicago ends with over 10 people shot, the countrywide outrage isn't as perceptible. Also, the Second Amendment does not equally apply to all Americans. Law-abiding minority citizens who have a legal firearm are still viewed as dangerous by society at large. Black civilians are not afforded the luxury of "exercising constitutional rights" when they have a legal firearm because of the stigmatization of being Black and armed. That didn't stop Black Americans from buying a lot more guns in 2020, though.

The fact is there are too many guns in America. There are nearly 400 million of them. For every 100 people in the country, there are over 120 guns. The United States is the only nation in the world where the number of guns is higher than the number of people. Though the actual number of illegal weapons is nearly impossible to know, many of the guns that started out as legal weapons find their way into the poor Black community. By the time they get to the hood—through trafficking and straw purchases—they have become illegal. You can look at law enforcement seizure efforts to get an idea of just how many illegal weapons are in these communities, a number that has grown since 2020, when firearm purchases went up. In 2021, police in Washington, DC, took over 2,400 illegal weapons off the streets. Halfway through 2022, there was a 54 percent increase in the number of guns the police recovered, compared with the first six months of 2021. The police in Chicago collected nearly 7,900 illegal guns in 2019, and that number went above 9,200 in 2020. What's even more disturbing about the case in Chicago is that during the height of the pandemic, there were fewer street and traffic stops happening but somehow the police collected even more guns than they had in the past. In an 11-month stretch in New York between 2021 and 2022, authorities seized over 1,400 illegal guns, which was a record number for the state police. The Milwaukee police have taken over 8,000 illegal firearms off the streets since 2020. These are just the ones that law enforcement is able to find. There are also ghost guns, which are homemade, untraceable firearms that are assembled from build-it-yourself kits or sometimes made with 3-D printers. Regular firearms, even illegal ones, are typically manufactured with a serial number that identifies the weapon and makes it easier for law enforcement to track it. Ghost guns don't have those serial numbers. Just as with other illegal weapons, it's difficult to know how many of them there are, but they've become more common.

Gun trafficking and straw purchases drive the daily community gun violence. Trafficking is when a weapon makes its way from a legal market to an illegal one. Usually, guns are trafficked across state lines, from a state with weak gun laws to a state with strong ones. It's not uncommon for traffickers in Georgia or South Carolina, two states with relatively weak laws, to traffic their guns to New York, a state with strong laws. The strong gun laws in states that struggle with gun violence are being undermined by the negligent laws in other states. A straw purchase is when someone buys a gun for somebody else—someone who likely can't get a legal firearm themselves. Because there is no federal antitrafficking law and each state has its own set of laws, there are major flaws in addressing the flow of illegal weapons. "There's some people who hear about gun regulations and enforcement of those regulations [and] they sort of poo poo that and say that's not getting at root causes," Professor Daniel Webster says. "I view it very differently. When you talk about root causes, the roots are public policy. When we're talking about laws and law enforcement that are upstream and preventing guns from getting into the wrong hands, that can decrease arrest and incarceration." If regulations and law enforcement do their jobs well, then fewer people will get their hands on a gun and the crimes they would commit can't happen, at least not with a firearm. But nationally we haven't addressed this, and during 2020 there was an increase in the number of people who procured guns, and more of these guns made it into the illegal market.

When it comes to the Constitution, though, there are people who are always going to support a citizen's right to own firearms. For example, the Supreme Court struck down a mainstay New York gun law in 2022 that said citizens needed to prove that they have a special need for protection if they want to carry a concealed firearm. With the law gone, it's now easier for New York residents to carry a gun outside their homes. This was the first time in over 10 years that the Supreme Court had ruled on a gun rights case. The case was brought by two men in New York who had been denied permits to carry firearms outside their homes and were backed by an NRA affiliate group in the state. Experts were concerned that the Supreme Court's decision would lead to similar laws being overturned in other states. This highlights the middle ground that needs to be found between the right to self-defense and commonsense gun laws.

Gun laws have to be part of the solution. The country needs to find a way to standardize firearm regulations, which lawmakers have already taken steps to do thanks to the 2022 Bipartisan Safer Communities Act. The bill includes the first-ever federal laws against interstate gun trafficking and straw purchases. Before the new act was implemented, federal background laws had a glaring (almost laughable) gap in that they allowed those who did not have a federal dealer's license to sell weapons without running any kind of background check. The new law covers that loophole and clarifies who needs to register as a firearm dealer. This will likely add more guns to the background check system. In an ideal scenario, background checks would be universal for all potential gun owners, something that pretty much all American citizens support. The hope is that background checks will become universal across all states and follow the same rules and regulations. Guns should only be able to be purchased one way: by going into a gun store, showing ID, filling out paperwork, and receiving a record showing that the gun is licensed to one name. That makes the person responsible for it. That way, going forward, it's easy to look up who owns what gun. So if it's stolen and used in a crime and the owner reports it stolen, there's a way to track it. On top of that, those under the age of 21 who want to purchase a gun would go through a more thorough background check.

Politicians, law enforcement, and others have advocated for these types of measures for decades. Lawmakers did a great job passing the Safer Communities Act, but they can't stop there. They need to find ways to continue to enhance federal gun laws. Another measure that would be helpful from a federal perspective is to come up with some type of gun dealer reform act—a way to monitor how gun stores and dealers are running their businesses. Most of the guns used in crimes in America can be traced to a small number—around 5 percent—of dealers. At the same time, it's hard for prosecutors to prove that a gun dealer willfully violated federal laws. So the more thorough and detailed these laws are, the more effective they can be when enforced.

It doesn't stop at the federal level. The states have work to do as well and can't rely on federal laws when prosecuting a major gun trafficker. Some states need to adopt stricter gun laws; others simply need to enforce the gun laws that they already have. It varies from place to place, but what typically makes a state's gun laws weak is if they lack things like universal background checks, gun trafficking penalties, open-carry regulations, concealed-carry laws, and community violence intervention funding. States with stronger regulations address all or most of these measures.

The Giffords Law Center to Prevent Gun Violence is one of the premier nonprofit organizations that promote stronger gun laws. Led by former US congresswoman Gabby Giffords—who survived an assassination attempt in 2011—the organization uses a wide array of experts, community leaders, lawyers, and former members of law enforcement and the gun industry for its work. The law center publishes detailed information about gun control and gun laws and assists politicians and public officials in their efforts to strengthen gun laws. In 2021 the Giffords Law Center ranked California, New Jersey, Connecticut, Hawaii, Massachusetts, New York, Maryland, Illinois, Rhode Island, and Washington as the 10 states with the strongest gun laws. The bottom 10 were Alaska, Arizona, Kentucky, South Dakota, Kansas, Mississippi, Missouri, Idaho, Wyoming, and Arkansas. These rankings are similar to those by other nonprofits that analyze state gun laws, including Everytown for Gun Safety, which does a lot of the same type of work as Giffords. Often, those who push back against the notion of strengthening gun laws point out that cities like Los Angeles, New York, Chicago, Baltimore, and Newark, which historically have struggled with gun violence, are in states that have "strong" gun laws. There's a simple explanation: they're close to states that have weaker gun laws, and the guns from these less strict states easily get into the states with stronger laws. But the states don't even have to be close to each other. Plenty of guns from Georgia, which is identified by Giffords as having weak gun laws, find their way into New York. The states with weak laws need to improve them, and the states with strong laws need to harshly enforce them. In the same way that lawmakers came together to pass the Bipartisan Safer Communities Act, state politicians have to find common ground. "We need stronger laws, whether those are at the state level or federal level. Policy changes will result in changes in how many guns are available on an underground market and, therefore, how frequently they're used in violent crime," Professor Webster explains. It's typically Republican-led states that block any attempts to strengthen gun laws.

What about mass shootings—or, more accurately, high-fatality mass shootings? Though they only account for about 1 percent of all gun violence deaths in the country, these incidents drive much of the national conversation on gun violence in America. It took the Uvalde mass shooting for lawmakers to put politics to the side and pass the Safer Communities Act. The public often asks why we can't stop high-fatality mass shootings. The problem is that they're so rare and often very random. This is why the focal point of those tragedies is the weapon used, which in almost all cases is an assault-style rifle or AR15. This is a discussion that (like every other discussion on gun laws) gets combative. Here's a simple fact, though: there is no way this country is going to be able to stop the deadly random mass shootings if almost anyone can go almost anywhere in the country and get their hands on the same kind of rifle that SWAT officers and soldiers use. Assault weapons make it too easy for someone to kill a high number of people. This might be a cynical way to look at it, but someone who is determined to kill a large group of people would not be able to do so with a shotgun. So in a sense, the goal is not to prevent harm, it's to prevent catastrophic harm. It's to prevent the Pulse nightclub shooting, the Las Vegas shooting, the Buffalo shooting, the El Paso shooting, and the Uvalde shooting. This all goes back to legislation: assault weapons need to be more heavily regulated. A lot of firearm experts like to use the analogy of cars. Before someone can drive a semitruck, they have to go through specific training and they have to get a commercial license. Why is that? Because a person can do a lot more damage with a commercial truck than they can with a regular car. We don't always require similar enhanced licensing processes for assault rifles. Lawmakers must find a way to better regulate and manage assault weapons and the people who can access them.

Can the country just ban assault weapons? We've tried it before. The last federal assault weapons ban came in 1994, partly in response to a mass shooting that happened in a San Francisco office building in 1993 where eight people were killed. President

Bill Clinton included the ban as part of his sweeping 1994 crime bill. The bill prohibited civilians from using or manufacturing certain assault weapons and types of ammunition. There's a lot of debate about how effective the weapons ban was. Critics say it didn't do much, as the inner-city gun violence continued. Many of the advocates for stronger gun laws say that high-fatality mass shootings did decrease during the period of the ban, and some researchers found a noteworthy reduction in mass shooting incidents when the ban was in place. However effective it might have been, the ban expired in 2004. Only six states and Washington, DC, have assault weapons bans—New Jersey, Maryland, Hawaii, Massachusetts, Connecticut, and California. Virginia and Minnesota regulate assault weapons but don't ban them. Some municipalities across the country also have their own set of bans in place. Just like other gun laws, assault weapons bans are easy to work around—someone can just get an assault weapon in another state or remove certain parts of a gun so it's not technically an assault weapon but has all the same characteristics. Another way the laws get skirted is through the use of a ghost gun or a ghost assault weapon. This goes back to the need for gun laws to be standardized, including those for assault weapons. Any federal assault weapons bans would need to set the groundwork for what's done at the state level.

The fight for stronger gun laws is a noble one and will be part of any long-term goal this country has to stop the daily crisis of firearm homicides, but these laws mean nothing without enforcement, and the Bureau of Alcohol, Tobacco, Firearms and Explosives (ATF) needs to be at the forefront of that enforcement. But when it comes to law enforcement agencies, not to mention federal ones, you'd be hard-pressed to find one that's been debilitated more than the ATF. Those who say that police departments have been defunded never seem to mention how funds have slowly been taken away from the ATF over the past 10 years. If there's going to be any hope of making sure these gun laws work, then the ATF will need to be a fully funded and healthy organization.

David Chipman is well aware of everything the ATF has gone through over the past 30 years. He grew up in Rochester, Michigan. He gained an interest in law enforcement at an early age and went to the American University in Washington, DC, to study criminal justice. While he was living in the nation's capital, Chipman was struck by the level of gun violence in the city. It wasn't going on where he lived on the northwest side of the city; it was centralized on the southwest side, the Black part of the city. The violence was not the only thing that caught his attention: it was also the public's reaction to it, or rather their indifference to it. During college, a professor of David's would quiz the class on something from the *Washington Post*, which forced the class to read it every day. David was startled by how the *Post* covered the violence. "It was just like one Black male shot with a gun, unknown address, it was like nothing. It was like what the fuck," David says. "It was such a revelation. It seemed weird that I was so close to this level of violence but still so far from it."

Already keen on being a part of law enforcement, David joined the ATF. The dangers of the drug war were the dominating narrative around the crime in the country. David didn't agree. "I wasn't concerned about the drug war. It didn't seem like drugs were the problem, it seemed like guns and violence was the problem," he says. His first posting was in Norfolk, Virginia, which David describes as "this iron pipeline of guns going up to New York." It was here that he learned all about gun trafficking and how it worked. He was also on the ground in Waco, Texas, during the 51-day siege in 1993 of the Branch Davidians compound that ended in the death of 76 people. Two years later, David was part of the team that responded to the Oklahoma City bombing, which was carried out by a domestic terrorist. In the mid-1990s, white extremist ideologies spread throughout the country. Many of the groups espousing these views were focused on arming themselves with as many weapons as they could, which is why the ATF was so interested in stopping them. Still, inner-city gun violence was a pressing issue. After the Oklahoma City bombing, David returned to his home state and worked in Detroit to fight the ongoing firearm crisis. He found out what a lot of others who are close to the issue of urban gun violence find: "We had this feeling that it was just a few people who were terrorizing these communities of color who didn't have the resources to get out. They were trapped." After spending years in the field, he made a move to headquarters to try to understand the politics of it all. "I needed to know what was providing the obstacles for us to do a better job," he says. He learned pretty quickly what was holding the ATF back: it was the politics. "I felt like we were doing a form of theater where it felt like we really weren't trying to prevent gun violence. We were trying to act more as a PR firm for the gun industry, which is not what I swore my oath to do," David explains. He left the ATF after that.

The woes of the agency can be traced back to the 1990s when the handling of two incidents—the Ruby Ridge standoff and the Waco siege—sparked widespread criticism of the agency and the federal government in general. The ATF was the focal point of that criticism, even in political circles. The growth of white nationalist and extremist groups helped frame the ATF as anti-American, which led to the development of the militia movement and opposition to firearm regulations. At the same time, the gun industry has made a concerted effort to stifle the agency and its leadership. The Tiahrt Amendment of 2003 disallows the ATF from publicly releasing any information from its firearms trace database. The ATF can only share that information with other law enforcement agencies or relevant prosecutors in a criminal case. These restrictions have made it difficult not only for the agency but for researchers and academics to have a better understanding of gun trafficking. That being said, what really did it in from a public perspective was the gun-walking scandal in the late 2000s. Between 2006 and 2011, ATF officials in Tucson and Phoenix allowed licensed gun dealers to sell weapons to illegal buyers, with the goal of tracking the weapons to drug cartels in Mexico. The operation was known as Fast and Furious and would become public after a border patrol agent was killed in 2010 in Arizona, near the Mexican border. Two assault rifles found at the scene were part of the ATF operation. In 2011, multiple ATF whistleblowers reported the operation to politicians, leading to an investigation. The agency's director at the time, Kenneth Melson, was reassigned and the US attorney in Arizona resigned. It was unclear who had knowledge of the scandal. Former attorney general Eric Holder initially said he didn't know anything about it, only to admit that he did during a Senate judiciary hearing.

Scandals are not uncommon for federal agencies, especially federal law enforcement agencies. The ATF also had issues with disproportionately targeting minorities when it expanded the use of stash house sting operations in the early 2000s. Those issues, along with other factors, have hurt the ATF's ability to do its job, which is partly to enforce the nation's gun laws. In addition, the agency has struggled with leadership since the director position became a Senate-confirmed job in 2006. For 15 years there had only been one director who was confirmed by the Senate: Byron Todd Jones, who led the agency from 2013 to 2015. The rest of the directors had been in an acting capacity. In April 2021, after years of working in the private sector, David became Biden's pick to lead the ATF. Unfortunately, he wouldn't get past his confirmation hearings. There was a coordinated effort by gun lobbyists and gun advocates to discredit him. He was framed as "antigun," and Senate Republicans weren't on board with him, even though anyone familiar with the gun laws and the ATF would tell you that David was probably the most qualified nominee in decades. "It became

clear to me that there were people who just did not want me leading the agency. I just had to accept that," David says. President
Biden pulled his nomination in September 2021.

Aside from its leadership issues, what also holds the ATF back
is its size. It's small compared with other federal law enforcement
agencies. It has around 5,000 full-time employees and a budget
of around $1 billion. For context, the FBI has 35,000 employees
and a $10 billion budget, the Drug Enforcement Administration
has 10,000 workers and a $3 billion budget, and US Immigration
and Customs Enforcement has 20,000 employees with an $8 bil-
lion budget. The ATF is even smaller than some big-city police
departments like the NYPD and the LAPD. Keep in mind, the ATF
is supposed to enforce federal gun laws nationally. So its 5,000
employees are supposed to enforce the laws for around 400 million guns. We can't expect federal laws to be effectively enforced
if the very agency that is in place to do it is as weak as the ATF is.
It needs consistent leadership. In July 2022 Biden's new pick to lead
the agency, Steve Dettelbach, was confirmed (though his confirmation process wasn't a cakewalk either). Dettelbach is a former
federal prosecutor and US attorney for the Northern District of
Ohio. He doesn't have the ATF experience that David Chipman
does, but he's said all the right things since he became the
director.

He previously spoke about the importance of gathering gun
crime intelligence, working with other law enforcement leaders,
being more preventive, and working with entire communities to
do prevention work. He also acknowledged that his agency is
smaller than some police departments but stressed the ATF is
going to have to do the best with what it has. "Look, I am not the
policy guy. I am the enforcement guy. Congress just came together
in a bipartisan way to give us more tools to try and deal with this
problem," Dettelbach said. "My job is to take what comes out of
Congress, the laws on the books, and make sure we're doing

everything we can to protect people." Hopefully, this director is there for the long haul, which should help the agency be more functional. He should become a consistent face in Congress and advocate there for his organization's fair share of the money. If the ATF is stronger, the agency can better enforce the nation's gun laws.

Dettelbach has put some action behind his words. For the first time in 20 years, the ATF released a detailed federal report on gun crimes in America in 2023. It showed how legal guns become illegal and how over a million guns were stolen between 2017 and 2021, among other information. The ATF also enacted a rule to go after ghost guns, announcing in the summer of 2022 that ghost guns must adhere to the same regulations as other guns. So if someone wants to buy a kit from a licensed retailer that has the parts to build a ghost gun, they'll have to go through a background check just as if they were buying a regular firearm. That's what the ATF should focus on. It's not realistic to attempt to take all guns away from people, so focusing on illegal ones and ghost guns is a good strategy for the agency. Local police departments can do their part as well if they're being strategic and targeting the violent criminals, who almost exclusively use illegal guns.

But none of this touches on the gun lobby and how effective it has been at stifling the progress of gun legislation over the past several decades. What exactly is the gun lobby? It's a broad term, but it essentially describes the efforts by gun groups to influence policy on gun laws and gun ownership. The NRA is the most well-known gun rights group but there are many others. These groups pay money to lobby lawmakers and support candidates who are opposed to strong gun control measures. One of their biggest lobbying successes was the Dicky Amendment, which was passed in 1996 as part of the 1997 Consolidated Appropriations Bill. The law states that "none of the funds made available for injury prevention and control at the Centers for Disease Control and Prevention

(CDC) may be used to advocate or promote gun control." This was after the CDC released a report in 1993 that showed guns in homes increased the risk of homicides in homes. While the amendment doesn't outright prohibit the funding of gun violence research, the CDC took that law as an implication that if it funded research that upsets or threatens the gun lobby, then it could lose significant funding. With that, 20 years went by without federal funding for gun violence research. This keeps the gun violence research community limited and small.

It's the gun lobby that was instrumental in stopping the confirmation of David Chipman and all the other potential leaders of the ATF until Dettelbach broke through. It may seem far removed from what happens on the ground, but the gun lobby plays a direct role in how gun violence affects poor communities. Its ability to keep stronger gun laws from being enacted has made it easier for guns to get into these neighborhoods. Those who operate in the gun lobby aren't even thinking about that, though. Their only goal is to sell as many guns as they can. Their message is that people need guns so they can protect themselves, and they lean on the Second Amendment as justification. What happens after the guns are sold doesn't matter to them. Because the gun lobby doesn't really answer to a branch of government or have any real oversight, addressing its impact is difficult. The Bipartisan Safer Communities Act is an important piece of gun legislation, but it's naive to think the gun lobby wasn't instrumental in undermining how much more effective it could have been. The NRA is nowhere near as powerful as it once was—thanks to a bevy of outside lawsuits and internal conflict among its ranks—but that just means other groups can fill the void.

In the summer of 2022, several gun rights groups in Colorado, a state that has decent gun laws, were successful in blocking an assault weapons ban that a county in the state had passed. They filed a lawsuit against the Boulder City Council after it passed a law to address gun violence, which included a ban on assault rifles. A judge sided with the gun group and cited the 2022 Supreme Court decision in New York as a justification for blocking the law. That's the kind of work that these local gun groups do all across the country. The efforts of those fighting for commonsense gun laws need to be just as widespread. That's not going to stop the gun lobby, but it'll balance out what it's doing.

Gun laws might be the trickiest factor of this entire issue, which is why it can feel removed from what's happening in the actual communities that have to deal with daily firearm violence. It involves high-level political players who couldn't be less concerned about the hood. The part community stakeholders harp on is how easy it is for people to get their hands on a gun. "We're not going upstream enough to figure out how all these guns are getting into the hands of these felons to begin with," Professor Webster explains. So it makes sense that the enforcement part of addressing gun laws is where a lot of attention should be. This does not diminish the efforts to make gun laws stronger. At some point, people with influence and power on the Republican side will need to step up and have some courage. It's the Republican Party that's holding up the passage of more sensible gun laws. Most American citizens support strong gun legislation. Politicians who don't cannot say they're serving the public. The country needs to find the balance between respecting a citizen's right to own a firearm and enacting commonsense firearm laws. Someone with a serious mental health issue should not be able to get their hands on a gun, regardless of what state they're in. At the same time, there are strong laws already on the books in different states and at the federal level that the ATF can enforce. If the agency can get the proper funding, leadership, and resources, it can better enforce the gun laws that are in place. While the agency grows, it can focus on the states from which guns are easily being trafficked. The politicians who push back against any type of reform for police departments need to shift that attention toward improving the law enforcement agency that is supposed to prevent people from getting their hands on these deadly weapons. Some of them can't because they're in the pocket of the gun lobby and it would be counterproductive. The ones who can (or have the courage to do so) could contribute greatly to this solution for gun violence. Because if the ATF could do its job better, then the cops who operate in the inner city wouldn't have as many guns to worry about.

7

The Community's Power

Anyone who talks to the adult version of Roy would find it hard to believe that he spent his teenage years as a stickup kid. What's even more surprising is learning that he went to prison for over 20 years. He's full of nothing but care and love today. Then again, as a violence prevention worker, his background makes him that much better at his job. Roy doesn't see the work he does today as a job, though—it's a calling to him. He feels like he went through everything he went through as a teenager and young adult so he could go back to his community and be part of the solution. The street cred that he has is just a tiny part of the work he does. It's certainly important—it allows him to get in front of certain people whom others can't have a conversation with—but the majority of the work is rooted in helping people heal so they can make better decisions, which in turn will reduce the turmoil in the community.

Whether as a violence interrupter or as a leader running interruption and youth programs, Roy has addressed the gun violence issue on a one-on-one basis. That means breaking up a conflict that has the potential to get violent, when someone is at their angriest and most volatile. It could mean getting in front of someone who has a gun and is ready to shoot someone else. Roy knows how dangerous the work is, but he calls it "absolutely necessary." What he really enjoys, though, are the community events, the ones where they can get as many people as possible involved. These get-togethers show just how much the residents care about gun violence and show the reach that Roy and his team have. For example, in the summer of 2021, a 26-year-old was shot and killed in their catchment area. The violence prevention team decided to organize a group response to the shooting, when members, volunteers, and anyone else who wants to be present goes to the spot where the shooting happened and talks to the community. Roy was the point man for this gathering.

Their office at the time was just off the major road that runs through several of the infamous Brooklyn neighborhoods like Crown Heights, Brownsville, and East New York. It was an active block with a handful of storefronts, corner stores, and people out and about. The foundation of the block is old-school Brooklyn, but the hints of gentrification are easy to find in the expensive coffee shops and brand-new vegan food spots that have started to appear. Inside, the office was small and cluttered. There were several desks set up, complemented by small office basketball hoops and a standing punching bag. These items were for the youth who worked there, but the adult workers would sneak in a jump shot or two.

In the back room of the office, the workers prepare for the event. Exuding a calm presence, Roy gathers all the necessary supplies. T-shirts, masks, snacks, a speaker, and a megaphone. None of this is new to him; he's done it plenty of times. He asks one of the youth workers to look for a bag of shirts in smaller sizes for kids. It's a friendly environment. All the workers mess with each other. Once all the supplies are set, the group heads out.

It's a comfortable summer day, not too hot. Roy leads a group of around 10 people. It's a mix of violence interrupters, youth workers, and volunteers. The shooting scene is about five blocks away from the office. As they walk, people greet them. They've built up a level of credibility in the neighborhood, among those in the streets and the everyday citizens. Even the police show them respect: a cop drives by the group as they walk and slows down to nod at them. They nod back.

They arrive on the corner where the shooting happened. It shouldn't be a surprise to anyone that Roy and his team are present. There are candles set up for the victim next to a corner store, which one of the workers takes note of: "There are candlelight memorials all over this city." The team starts to engage with the community. They take turns on the megaphone. "My team is out here today to take a stand. A stand for our community, a stand for our youth. As I stand here on this block, it saddens me because I know there are a lot of kids that live on this block and I don't see not one out here playing. In the middle of the summertime, the children don't even feel like they can come outside and play in this community," one of the violence interrupters says. Another one takes the megaphone to make a different point. "I can most guarantee you that's your brother, that's a friend, somebody you grew up with. They know your mother, grandmother probably, uncle, aunt, and we out here killing each other," the interrupter says. "What are we doing? When is enough enough?"

As they pass the megaphone around, some residents stand and watch, affirming the words said. Some of the workers speak individually with people who walk by or stop to see what's going on. Even for the people who aren't out watching the event, it's hard to imagine they can't hear the megaphone from inside their homes on the block. The workers aren't shouting at people; they're not being disrespectful. They speak clearly but firmly. They know the community needs to hear this. Even if people aren't acknowledging them, they believe the message is being received in some way. "We need unity," another interrupter declares. There aren't a ton of people present but it's a lively scene. One resident, an older gentleman who's probably seen a fair amount of violence in the community, has a spirited debate with one of the workers. He says these kids (the ones doing the shootings) are too far gone and just need to be locked up. "What can we really do for them?" he asks one of the interrupters. The violence prevention worker doesn't agree with this but continues the debate with the resident. It's spirited but respectful. The worker says he has a responsibility to these kids because he was one of them, and if he could make a change in his life, then maybe the kids would be able to do the same. The elderly man says most of the kids will end up dead if they don't get locked up. He says the violence interrupter was "fortunate" to come back home from prison. As all of this goes on, a cop car is parked across the street from the event, almost as if they were assigned this corner because of the shooting. One of the officers gets out of the car and observes the gathering.

After about 45 minutes, the team walks back to their office. This event didn't bring out the largest group of people, but it was still important for the team to organize the response. "We know the word about us spreads. When things happen, it's gotten to the point where people are looking for us and wondering how we're going to respond and help out," Roy says. It could be a simple event like this local response or a bigger one like the march across the Brooklyn Bridge they organized in the summer of 2022. It was for a Brooklyn man who was killed in 2020. His mother and other mothers who lost children to gun violence were present. Over 30 people attended. Some reporters showed up as well.

Before this event starts, the group waits for the mothers to arrive in a Brooklyn park with the New York City skyline in the background. Roy and the workers discuss mundane topics as they wait, like their health insurance and the number of groups texts they're in. These guys do vital work for the city, but they're still just regular coworkers who are comfortable and carefree around one another.

Before the march starts, the mother gives a quick speech, thanking those in attendance and the organizers as well. "We can't go nowhere without God," she declares. In that spirit, a pastor gives a prayer before they all walk across the bridge. As they march, they chant. "Man up, not down"; "We all we need, we all we got." Some hold signs with other phrases and pictures of gun violence victims. As they walk, onlookers take notice of the chants and signs. Many of them nod in agreement, even the tourists who don't live in the city.

Roy and his group don't just get people together after a tragedy. They have plenty of fun and engaging happenings for community members. Like the youth basketball league they're involved in over the summers. During the championship game in 2022, a popular Brooklyn park is filled with players, spectators, families, DJs, and those just passing by. Cookout food is provided to attendees. One of the championship games features teens around 16 and 17 years old. It's a lively and competitive game. Elbows flying, hard fouls, guys yelling "and one" after a layup (even if they missed it and didn't get a foul call), and of course some aggressive dunks. Players talk trash to each other: "he food," "that's a bucket," "pressure everything," and "this nigga can't guard me." It's classic New York City streetball, physical and intense, but it doesn't go past the game itself. That's because the organizations that put this together are there. It's a controlled environment. "It's just something to get the community together during the summer months," Roy says.

Violence interruption, community responses to shootings, and community gatherings: these are all the ways Roy takes responsibility for what is happening in his neighborhood. This is how he combats the gun violence that has plagued his hometown since he was a kid. Regardless of what the police, the government, or anyone outside the area is doing, Roy knows the community itself has a pivotal part in all of this. "The community absolutely has a role because it impacts them. What that role looks like? It varies from person to person but my hope is that their role would be centered around connecting with organizations and community members to raise their voice against gun violence," Roy says. That's certainly one way for individuals in the affected neighborhoods to take part in addressing the problem, but there are plenty of other ways for people to play a role. One of the more ignorant statements that those on the outside make about gun violence is that folks who live in the hood don't care about it—that they only care about gun violence when the triggerman is a police officer. That's far from the truth. Most people who live in these neighborhoods care deeply about the problem. Even beyond that, many of them don't want to wait on the government or the police to fix it, which creates a bit of tension between different factions within the communities that work to address the issue. "We are failing our community and we have to do better. It takes the community as well. It takes participation from the community as well to end the gun violence in our own communities," one violence interrupter says during the August 2021 shooting response.

The everyday law-abiding citizen isn't causing the problem, so do they have to be out like Roy, risking their lives to stop the next shooting? Absolutely not. In all honesty, violence interruption and outreach work is not something a lot of people should be doing. There shouldn't be hundreds and hundreds of violence interrupters. The work is hard and dangerous. It should only be for those who are truly committed to it and know the risks. Regular citizens can get involved with other community organizations, and they can make appearances at rallies and gatherings, but they don't even have to do that. They can simply look out for their kids and ensure they aren't committing crimes in the streets. The Black parents in the hood who have a strong lid over what their children are doing may not realize it, but they're helping to stop the cycle. They're keeping their kids away from the guns and the drugs and the temptation that's on the streets.

Then you have the people who take more proactive actions, ones who weren't in the streets at all but still feel responsible for addressing the problems that go on. People like Erica Ford in New York, Tamar Manasseh in Chicago, Cheryl Riviere in Baltimore, Pastor Donovan Price in Chicago, and Guy Burney in Youngstown. The list goes on and on. These are people who see the issues plaguing their community, including gun violence. They could just keep their heads down and live their lives, but they're taking responsibility for what's happening and working to try to fix it. So what about the ones who are already in the streets, the ones who don't step outside without a gun? This is when it gets complicated. Conventional wisdom says for them to just put the gun down. That's what most old-school people will say. "All of this would stop if people just put the weapon down." Yes, that's true, and in a perfect world everyone would do that.

In reality, though, a lot of these guys feel like they need a gun to protect themselves. Not the ones who shoot up blocks indiscriminately while trying to hit a rival; the guys who are out in the streets but not necessarily active in them. It's about protection. They don't want to rely on the police for safety, because they feel that should be their own responsibility. So they consistently have a gun on them. If you told them to put the gun down, their response would be something like, "If everyone else puts theirs down, I will." It's a tricky dynamic. Davante Griffin, the Atlanta man who was shot in his own room after a home invasion in 2021, has thought about this. Often, when he's out in public, he has his gun on him. He just never knows when something is going to happen. Even when his son is in the backseat, Davante drives with the gun right on his lap. "No matter who you are, somebody think you sweet. You could be the biggest toughest nigga in the world. Somebody thinks you can get got," he explains. Aside from his own personal experience in 2021, an incident that serves as a reminder for him involved a friend of his (the same friend who was shot five times when Davante's house was broken into). Sometime after the shoot-out at Davante's house, this friend was in a gas station store. Two people (who Davante believes might have recognized his friend from a previous encounter) came into the store and positioned themselves to ambush Davante's friend. He quickly picked up on the situation, took out his gun, and started firing at them. They ran out of the store. One of them was hit, but they got in their car and drove off.

Davante doesn't want to take any chances when it comes to his life and his son's life. He wishes he didn't have to carry a gun in public, but that's not his reality. What he can do, though, is be accountable for his own actions, something he takes very seriously. Take the home invasion. There was a period of time after he healed when he felt like he knew who might have been responsible for it. He wasn't 100 percent sure, but he had a pretty good idea. Part of him wanted revenge—he wanted to go out and kill the person he believed was responsible for the attack. He felt like he had every right to retaliate. His son had been in the house just before the gunmen broke in. If this person was so willing to set up Davante and his family, then he must've known that there might be some retribution if it didn't go through. But as Davante thought it through, it just made no sense to do something about it. "What would really come out of that? A bunch of retaliation. Everybody knows that there's consequences behind it. You can do certain shit but then it comes back on you," Davante says. "Me going out here and killing somebody—like, I got a son. If I got to go to jail, how am I going to tell him what not to do if I'm in jail? There would be so much that he goes through without me. I don't want him to have to go through that." That's a level of maturity and foresight that a lot of people involved in the streets don't typically have. Talk to anybody who works in the hood (police, community leaders, activists, regular residents) and they'll tell you that many of the shootings that happen are driven by retaliation for something another person did or was believed to have done. They're done in the heat of the moment and come out of anger. That often leads to the death of innocent civilians like people at barbecues or someone who happens to be walking by a few guys in the middle of a conflict with someone else.

In the case of Davante, he made a conscious decision to just leave it alone. Does it hurt his ego or make him feel like less of a man? Maybe, but to him being a real man is being there for his son at all costs. Roy calls that type of decision "powerful." "I think that's a value-based and knowledge-based decision because you're thinking about your child, your family, and the repercussions," Roy says. "That's a difficult decision to make because when you're in the streets all you're thinking about is getting some get back." Roy thinks such cases should definitely be held out as an example for others. Just look at Atlanta alone, which had 160 homicides in 2021. There's no way to know how many of these were in retaliation for something else, but hypothetically, what if 50 percent of the people who shot and killed someone as an act of revenge for something else had instead made the same decision Davante did that year after he was shot? What would that do to the homicide numbers? Some people who are in gangs feel like if they don't retaliate then they'll end up getting killed themselves. So they may feel like they can't take the same stance as Davante because they're walking around with a target on their back. This is why the solutions to gun violence have to be comprehensive. Situations like this are where the police and community organizations should step in. But there is something to be said for personal responsibility.

A person can only control their actions. Self-defense is necessary and people should always be ready to protect themselves as best they can. But someone should not go out of their way to shoot someone else. Ideally, everyone would just put their guns down, but the way Davante moves is probably the best kind of compromise for people who are in the streets, at least until other actions to address gun violence are implemented properly. "Gun violence is the tip of the iceberg. There are other issues that are driving people to reach the type of mindset for wanting to hurt others," Roy says.

That's absolutely true, but it does not negate the personal responsibility of people in the community. What's interesting is that it's almost frowned upon to make this point about inner-city neighborhoods that struggle with gun violence, especially when it's framed in a way that ignores the other systemic and societal issues. The people who actually live in these communities don't tend to feel that way, though. They know multiple things can be true. It's necessary for people to have some responsibility for what's going on in the areas they live in, just like it's necessary for the other issues to be addressed. Take Baltimore, for example. The city has been clocking over 300 murders a year since 2015. No one cares more about these murders than the people who actually live in the community. Not the police apologists who defend law enforcement from the safety and comfort of their homes: it's the residents who get up every day and have to walk by police tape and bullet holes in the windows. The part that's missed by people who look at the issue from the outside is that most of the efforts in the community to make change come from those who were part of the streets. The self-accountability that's preached comes from folks who were committing the crimes. It comes from people like Antoin Quarles, a Baltimore native who spent nearly two decades behind bars for various crimes. Now he runs a group called HOPE Baltimore, which works with individuals who have recently been released from prison, helping them find jobs and housing and get reacclimated to life outside. It's a small organization but it's been an important group for the people it's helped since starting in 2016. "I remember coming home and not knowing how I was going to live and when I saw other people coming home and needing resources it gave me a passion," Antoin says. "I wanted to be part of something, I wanted to build something for my community." Antoin built the organization piece by piece. That's what personal responsibility looks like: a man who made mistakes, recognizes those mistakes, and not only works to change but helps others as well.

HOPE usually has meetings every Tuesday night, at the Emmanuel Episcopal Church in Baltimore, about a mile north of the Inner Harbor. During one meeting in the summer of 2022, a handful of members attend. They gather in a side room in the church. The room is nice, dimly lit and spacious. Couches and chairs are spread around. The space has an old feel to it, which makes sense because the church was built in 1854. The members start to gather inside the room, maybe 12 of them. All of them are Black men and all of them have spent time in prison. They act familiar with each other as they laugh and argue about the food. It's pizza. Whatever these men may have done in the past, today they're as respectful and welcoming as any other members of society. Before they get into the real discussion, they hang out for a bit. One of them talks about Mike Evans, the man who created the popular 1970s Black sitcom *Good Times*. He says he wishes there were more Black shows like that on TV today. Others agree.

At 6:41, the meeting begins. They discuss things going on in their personal lives, their communities, how they can get help, and how they can help each other. One person makes a point about politicians needing to step up more in helping organizations like HOPE. "They're around when they running office but once they get in office, they disappear," he says. The conversation shifts to a lack of resources for them to take advantage of, and some observe that there are more resources available for women. But another member pushes back. "If you gotta get two jobs, get two jobs," he says. This same person says that regardless of the circumstances, "we create our own conditions. We got to take our own accountability." He knows that can be hard and explains that he used to be filled with a large amount of hate and it took him years to get rid of it. "You gotta love yourself more than you hate someone else. Hate becomes a prison." This sparks a bevy of responses from others, who for the most part agree. "Don't let the environment dictate your actions," another member says. He stresses that there is a difference between "being a man in the hood and just being a man." Another person talks about losing two friends to gun violence in the past week; one of them was a "citizen" and wasn't in the streets. He agrees overall with the need for responsibility but also says that the youth have so much working against them. "That's why we gotta step up," one man says. "It's up to us." It's a spirited meeting, with a lot of passion and strong points being made by everyone who speaks.

The point about Black men stepping up is crucial. It's a perspective that can be found in many of the neighborhoods that struggle with gun violence. Like everything around the issue, it needs the proper context. Black men are without a doubt the easiest target for law enforcement in this country. Though the numbers have steadily declined over the past decade, for every 100,000 Black citizens, around 938 are in prison, according to 2020 data from the Bureau of Justice Statistics. It's less than 200 for white people, though they make up 75 percent of the US population and Black people hover around 13 percent. With prison populations being over 93 percent male, it's easy to deduce who's locked up. It's also easy to deduce how those prisons were filled up with Black males. During the late 1980s and '90s, when mass incarceration was an emphasis for the government at the city, state, and federal levels, the weight of that emphasis fell on Black men and on the families in the communities that were targeted. "Mass incarcer-

ation killed us. It destroyed the family, it destroyed the community," Tyrone Parker of Washington, DC, says. Now Black men are
also the primary victims of gun violence, so it's a difficult dynamic
to examine. There's enough anecdotal evidence of how many
young Black kids grow up without a father in their lives. Whatever
reason someone wants to point to, that has fractured the Black
community and made an issue like gun violence more damaging.
"There is certainly a need for Black men and Black fathers to
take a more assertive role in their communities," Roy says. "We're
supposed to be the ones who represent the strength of the family
and the community, and in a lot of ways that's been broken in
the Black community." In no uncertain terms, Roy believes if
more Black men were in their kids' lives, it would be a huge help
for an issue like gun violence. Pastor Price, the Chicago activist
who travels to shooting scenes in the city and provides prayer
and services for the victim's family in the aftermath of the incident, sees the importance of Black male role models as well. He
recalls having a conversation with a 12-year-old who was a known
shooter and asking him, "How did you get to this point?" The kid
gave him a cold look and said, "I ain't never had a dad to disap-
point." The pastor had to stop and think about that. This topic
can be complicated to discuss candidly because it can be viewed
as an attack against the Black women who have the heavy burden of taking charge in the Black community. It's not an attack on
them, though; it's more about Black men needing to step up and
do their part in addressing the issues.

Anthony Jones feels strongly about the role of Black men in the
community. He was raised on the east side of Youngstown, Ohio.
He grew up in a two-parent household, but this was Youngstown
in the 1990s, so he was around everything. "We were surrounded
by gang-affiliated folks," Anthony says. "Every side of town had
affiliations." At that time, Youngstown had one of the highest
murder rates in the country. What made it worse was that there

wasn't much to do in Youngstown but get involved with gangs. Anthony credits his parents with keeping him away from the streets, though. It would have been easy for him to fall into the trap, but his father took his responsibility to another level. Anthony was in one of the only two-parent households in his neighborhood. His father had a lot of respect in the community. "There were 16 kids in our neighborhood around my age, 3 of us had fathers," Anthony recalls. "My dad was the neighborhood dad." Anthony's father didn't just raise and look after his own son, he was doing that for other kids in the neighborhood as well. So much so that Anthony resented it as a kid. He wondered why his father took so much time to help these other kids. Of course, he was there for his own son, but he also made a concerted effort to be a role model and father figure to others. "It wasn't until I got older that I understood," Anthony says today.

Most in the community are aware of why the presence of Black male role models is an issue. It's not an accident that Black men were out of the picture for a lot of Black families starting in the 1990s. "It was systemic. They locked Black men up," Anthony says. Should the expectation be that all Black fathers take responsibility for the kids in their neighborhoods who unfortunately don't have a male figure in their life? No. What Anthony's father did was extraordinary but it's not the norm. What should be the norm is more connectivity in these communities. Fathers, mothers, leaders—it doesn't matter who the person is. It's about there being more kinship in the neighborhoods that struggle with gun violence, more people looking out for one another, more parents being on the lookout for other kids. When community groups have events, it's about more people showing up. "People want to help. They want their neighborhoods improved," a Washington, DC, violence interrupter says. That's the goal of all of this. People in the hood feel like their communities are not united. It's easier in small cities like Youngstown for such kinship to take form, but

Anthony says COVID-19 put a dent in some of those efforts. The pandemic prompted an increase in crime in the city, like in other cities. One thing that stood out to Anthony, though, was the local rap music in the city. "The music influenced a lot of what was going on. Plus the artists making the music are so young," he says. "They're talking about shooting a gun and feeling the power of it. That's what they're glorifying."

It would be ignorant to blame rap music for the persistent gun violence that happens in the poor Black community, but it would also be irresponsible to not mention it in this context. The connection between rap music and the streets is well documented. Rap music is not a monolith, but its reputation is that it's only about crime, violence, drugs, misogyny, and immorality. Today, though, rap music is pop culture. It's one of the most popular and mainstream forms of music in the country, and its impact goes beyond the Black neighborhoods where it originated. But that mainstream popularity doesn't negate its origins. Because of its connection to the streets, a lot of the artists have strong ties to the disenfranchised communities they came from. The music means a lot more in the Black community than anywhere else. This is especially apparent when young rap artists are gunned down. An unsettling number of rappers have been killed as a result of gun violence in recent times. These aren't just local rappers who only have buzz in their neighborhoods—real stars have lost their lives. The part that's so heartbreaking is how young some of them are. XXX Tentacion was 20 when he was killed in Florida in 2018. Pop Smoke, a rising Brooklyn rapper, was also 20 when he was shot and killed in Los Angeles. King Von was 26 when he was killed. Takeoff, a member of the iconic Migos group, was 28. Nipsey Hussle was 33. All of these guys were stars, some of the biggest stars in the genre.

There's an age-old debate about the impact rap music has on the Black community and why the community allows it to be a mainstay. That debate isn't going anywhere. The divide is usually across age groups. Music is supposed to be a form of entertainment. Nothing more. The argument that's made in defense of rap music compares it to movies about crime and violence. People who love crime movies aren't getting involved in criminal activity. Actors who act in those movies aren't getting gunned down at a disproportionate rate. The other side argues that rap music has created a destructive culture in the Black community. It's not as simple as either side makes it out to be, but there are probably bits of truth to both. What's happened since the late 2010s around hip-hop music is a little different, though, because the most popular subgenre of rap, drill music, has a much more direct connection to the streets. A lot of these artists are in gangs and discuss real disagreements and conflicts in their music. They name-drop someone who was actually killed or threaten to kill a real enemy. It's gotten to the point where politicians have targeted drill music and made attempts to censor it or use law enforcement to go after the artists involved. For the most part, rappers are speaking hypothetically. Yes, rappers in the past had conflicts with other rappers and went at each other on records and in public, but what's happening in the drill music scene is a bit different. These are gang members and street kids who are becoming rappers. In the music, they're cursing dead rivals and it gets very personal. Rap beefs don't typically end in bloodshed. Rapping is competitive, but it's supposed to be kept in the music. A lot of the drill rappers, however, are treating their rap conflicts like real street conflicts. "This is what happens when you mix music with the streets. The line becomes blurred," Davante says.

So what is the community's responsibility for rap music? On the positive side, rap music gives people in the hood hope. The belief is that people can become successful through music. There's a serious question as to whether that should be a focal point in these neighborhoods (ask most of the adults in the hood and they'll say no), but it's viewed by the youth as something to get you out of your environment. The negative side is simple: there is a danger that the youth will enact the criminality described by rappers in the streets. "Parents need to tell their kids that this is not real. The police are real, laws are real. The music is not real," Pastor Price says. A lot of the most successful rappers who are talking about criminal activity aren't actually engaging in it. Tragically, the ones who do often end up in jail or dead. This is not to target rap music as the cause of something like gun violence. Again, daily shootings are the result of a lot of different factors. Still, rap music has a clear presence in the communities that struggle most with gun violence, and pretending it doesn't play a role is insincere.

Then there's the issue of trust, which is difficult to overcome. People in the hood have little trust in the government. Not just in something like the police but in hospitals, social services, and local politicians. This is where community leaders come into play. The church pastors have connections to those entities. They need to find a way to bridge that gap. Of course, the responsibility isn't all on the community to do this, but they have to be open to working with the government. While parts of the system need to be adjusted (whether through investment or more strategy on the part of law enforcement), people need to find a way to have more faith in those systems and work with them in the efforts to fix the problem. On the policing side, this comes down to the "no-snitching" rule. If the police do a better job of protecting and trusting residents who bravely step up and tell them something, then more residents will be willing to come forward. But both sides need to trust each other for that to happen.

Data are important, and many of these points aren't rooted in data or real evidence. They are more about feelings and perspectives. Those who live in struggling areas know that there is truth to all of this. Gun violence—all crime, for that matter—is sometimes seen as the defining characteristic of the Black community.

It's unfair and unfortunate because it's not true. These are places where people grow up, start families, start businesses, and live fulfilling lives. So when a prominent Black person proposes this idea of personal responsibility or accountability in a public forum as a way to handle the problem, they're usually criticized for playing the "respectability politics" game.

Someone like Delano Squires gets targeted for that by his critics. Delano was born and raised in a blue-collar family in Queens, New York City. He's familiar with what goes on in the hood. He recalls the first time he ever drove on the highway. It was the day that Patrick Dorismond—a Black man who was shot and killed by an undercover cop in 2000 in New York City—was buried. Delano was in the car with his dad, headed to a bowling alley in Brooklyn. As he got onto the highway, protesters were out on the streets, confronting the police. "I saw people coming around the corner, throwing bricks, rocks at the police," Delano says. "My dad was like, 'We gotta get outta here.' I gunned our Pontiac 6000 onto the highway."

After attending college and grad school, Delano worked in the local Washington, DC, government for 14 years, primarily to address the digital divide in the city. "When we first got started, about 40 percent of DC households did not have internet connection. We promoted low-cost home internet service, provided tech for low-income residents," Delano says. "We focused our efforts on populations that were most likely to be offline, disconnected, or did not use tech. A lot of low-income families, older adults, and citizens returning home from prison."

His final year with the DC government was in the city's Office of Gun Violence Prevention in 2021, as a resident liaison. He spoke with concerned community members about the surge in gun violence and explained the city's plan to address the problem. "I had a front-seat view of the victims and the perpetrators of gun violence in the city," he says.

Delano doesn't have any revolutionary opinions about gun violence. He sees the chaos that happened in 2020 as a contributing factor to the surge. He argues that "when the response to violent crime is we need more restraints on law enforcement, you're sending the wrong signals." He believes that mediation, intervention, and strategic policing can all address the problem. "I think targeting specific communities, specific crews, having people who can go there and talk to guys who are most likely to engage in retaliation shootings is helpful," he says. There's nothing out of the ordinary about Delano's opinions on gun violence. But they receive a bit more attention because he's also a commentator and cultural critic. He makes a lot of media appearances and writes columns, mainly on issues on family, gender, faith, and marriage.

Delano is a staunch believer in the nuclear family and is more than comfortable sharing his thoughts about it publicly. This is why he gets a lot of pushback from other notable Black commentators who are more on the liberal side. The issue of the family ties to gun violence in the hood, but there is a divide within the Black community on it. Everyone knows gun violence is a problem and Black people care deeply about it. The differences come into play when the discussion turns to accountability and who has that responsibility. When someone like Delano talks more about personal responsibility and the role of families in these communities, it's looked at by others as a way to ignore the more systemic issues.

But Delano is not alone. Folks in these communities always bring up accountability when they talk about gun violence. Listen to what the violence prevention workers say at their rallies and gatherings. Listen to the pastors who handle the funerals for victims of gun violence. Talk to the community leaders and get their thoughts. Talk to everyday citizens who are just trying to live their lives. They all say people need to take ownership for their actions.

The emphasis is on the Black community because that's where most of the gun violence happens.

That does not negate the other factors. Poverty still exists, guns are still in the community, and the police still struggle to handle the problem. "It starts with us, though. It has to matter to us more than anyone else," Anthony says. That's the irony of this issue. Black people in the hood care. They care more than most. The narrative that they don't is a lie told to paint a picture of complete indifference, like Black people in the hood are not capable of caring about themselves and need white people from the outside to save them because they're inherently violent and evil. If you visit any inner-city community, you'll see the number of sermons, candlelight vigils, and programs that are put together in response to all the violence. These are organized by the people who actually live there.

The folks who live in these communities are some of the strongest and most resilient people in the country. They're battling a government system that doesn't care about them. Citizens have to find a way to maneuver through neighborhoods that are plagued with guns and drugs and every other reason to fail. Just as they want the systems around them to step up, they want to see the people around them step up as well. Most people in the hood are not criminals. It's a small percentage who make it bad for everyone. The families of Roy, Davante, Anthony, and Delano all had high expectations of their kids. No one is saying this is the fault of inner-city residents. They didn't ask for their neighborhoods to be marginalized and disenfranchised for generations. That's just how it is, and many of the people on the ground in these places want to see their neighbors refuse to let these circumstances define them.

Davante puts a button on it: "We can be better. We can do so much more than anyone thinks we can."

PART III

The (Hopeful) Future

8

Where the Evidence Works

"Yo, you hear all that that's going on outside?" a colleague asked Roy while he was in his organization's office over the summer of 2022. Roy was on the phone so he wasn't paying attention to outside, but when he did he saw two men arguing. It didn't look like it was going to end well, so he went outside. "Yo, that's my bike. What you doing with my bike?," one of the men said to the other. The man who had the bike wasn't giving it up—in fact, he got on the bike and rode off. The other man chased after him, on a different bike. Roy saw all of this happen in real time and was walking over to try to intervene but they both dipped out. Still, Roy kept his ears open about it. Later on that day, Roy saw the guy who had wanted his bike back. He had it now. Roy approached the man. "It's kind of like an intervention but more so on the other side of it," Roy explains, meaning he's addressing it after the fact. He tells the man he saw what happened. "Yo, you seen that?" the man asks, almost looking for affirmation that what the other guy did was wrong. "Yeah, I was coming over but ya'll rode off with the bikes. What happened?" Roy asked. The man explained that a few days prior he had gone inside a store on this very block and left his bike outside, and when he came back the bike was gone. Today, though, the man who took it came back to the block. "This guy back over here with my bike. He stole my bike and he's back over here with it," the man says, wondering how this person could be clueless enough to come back to the same spot where he took the bike.

After this man confronted him, he ended up chasing him all the way to Brownsville, about two miles east of where the bike was taken. He got the bike back without any issues. Roy thought this was the end of the story, and it was noteworthy that it ended without any violence. In the hood, these conflicts go bad a lot more often than they go well. But this man was still angry about it. "If I see him again I'ma shoot him," he said to Roy. "He lucky I ain't have anything on me," he said. Turns out Roy would have to do some work on this incident. He tried to reason with him. "First of all, you got your bike back. It didn't even lead into a fistfight right there." He asked him what sense there would be in going back at him after he already got the bike back. "Nah, man, it's the principle—like, he lucky I ain't had nothing on me," he said. Roy tried to play this out for the man. "If you go at him and, God forbid, he gets killed, he's dead and your life is over after that," Roy said. He could see the wheels turning in the guy's head. It's like he hadn't really thought everything through, he was just heated. After he posed the question, Roy could see that it weighed on the man a bit. He wasn't pushing back like he had been when Roy first approached him. He ended up agreeing with Roy and said he would leave it alone. Roy was glad this situation took care of itself in a way, but he wishes he had been able to step in before the chase happened. "It played out in a way where no one was hurt. I'm glad I was able to speak a little sense into him, though," Roy says.

Was that the most dangerous type of situation a violence interrupter could be in? Of course not, but it shows the diligence that workers like Roy have. From the outside looking in, this incident could be viewed as one that did not require Roy to get involved, especially after the fact when the two rode away. This wasn't a gang conflict or a shooting incident where information needed to be gathered. But what if later on that man ended up killing the guy who stole his bike? Did Roy's conversation with him truly sway him from doing it? It certainly couldn't have hurt the situation. Roy is someone familiar with the streets who is keeping an eye on things and offering compassion and intervention. This is why community-based solutions are pivotal to solving this problem.

Sometimes there are higher stakes in the situations that these workers deal with. Over the summer of 2022, Sharod, a violence interrupter in the East New York neighborhood of Brooklyn, was circling a conflict going on between two men. He learned about a fight that had occurred between the two over some disrespect. Street guys have zero tolerance for disrespect. Sharod intervened and spoke with each man separately. He wanted them to let the situation go. It seemed like his words were convincing and they agreed to drop it. A few days went by, however, and Sharod heard through others that one of the men had not let it go. In fact, it was now a life-or-death situation. One of the men was going to try to kill the other. His plan was to shoot him while he was playing basketball near the Pink Houses, a notorious public housing complex in Brooklyn. Violence interrupters can't go to the police, not if they want to have any credibility with people in the community. So Sharod decided to warn the man who was going to be a potential victim. "I told him to stay off the streets and keep his eyes open while I go and talk to the other guy again," Sharod says. This was dangerous, but it is what these workers do. He got in touch with the potential shooter. They met at the park where he planned to do the shooting. Sharod begged the man not to do it. "I just pleaded with the brother. I told him this was pointless and that it wouldn't solve anything," he says. Then he made a proposal: What if he could get the two men to meet up in a public spot, with no guns, and just hash out their issues? If they had to fistfight for a second, so be it, but he wanted this resolved without anyone's death. The potential shooter agreed. A day or so later, they met up. Sharod didn't take any chances: he had a few other workers there with him. They made sure neither one of the men had a gun on him. It was a charged conversation. The men cursed at each other, and it felt like it was a couple of seconds away from getting physical. It turns out their disagreement was over a comment one of the men made about the other's sister. In the end, the two agreed to stay out of each other's way and not interact anymore. Sharod was relieved. He felt like this one almost slipped through his hands but he stopped it from getting violent. This sort of work is not perfect, but it's a useful tool.

This can be seen in Racine County, Wisconsin, which is about 23 miles south of Milwaukee. Nakeyda Haymer began volunteering as a violence interrupter in the county after her older brother was shot and killed in 2017. Like others who lose a family member to violence, she was angry and wanted revenge. "When you lose somebody it does hurt, you do have a void, but there's ways to fill that void instead of violence and retaliating you can build things positively and create a purpose and passion from the pain," Nakeyda previously said. She volunteered with the Voices of Black Mothers United group in the county and would go to the scene where a shooting happened, find the family of the victim, and console them. She provided them with comfort and tried to talk them out of any vengeful actions. Her efforts caught the eye of the county government and she was named the county's first violent crime reduction coordinator in 2022. The work of the community is important, and it's also important for that work to be supported by the local government.

There is no perfect solution to gun violence, but Roy, Nakeyda, and Sharod show the value of their work. It isn't theoretical, it's practical. The same goes for the other proposed solutions to gun violence. Are any of them going to be immaculate? No, but if the proper work is done when these solutions are applied, they can be effective. The same goes for good policing. When police are actually strategic and focus on the right things in these neighborhoods, they have positive impacts. Like in St. Louis, when detectives worked diligently to solve a couple of murders that happened in 2022. When they arrested a suspect, they connected him to two shootings from the prior year. That was the result of strategic police work. It took a while to put it all together, but that's what is required to do effective policing.

This can also be seen in an incident that occurred in Minneapolis a few years ago. Detective Aaron Clayton had spent years building relationships with people as a beat cop in the South Minneapolis area. He was someone whom residents trusted simply because he treated them fairly and with respect. Though he was no longer a beat cop in the area, he maintained a connection with the people he spent years speaking to. When a gang member was shot and killed in South Minneapolis in 2019, the investigation followed all the usual patterns that inner-city homicide cases do. The two detectives on the case couldn't get anyone to speak with them. No witnesses came forward to share information. The detectives reached a dead end almost immediately after the shooting happened. They were stuck, but they knew Aaron had connections to the area so they went to him for help. He put them in touch with a community leader who tends to be more plugged into what's going on in the streets.

This person was able to provide the detectives with more context about the shooting, but they still had no real leads. Frustrated, they were ready to move on. Aaron could have let it go too. He wasn't on the case. It meant nothing to his record, but he wanted to help as much as he could. Because he had spent years gaining familiarity with the neighborhood, he was able to work on certain angles and get more information. He found out that someone had not only been bragging about the shooting but also showing off the gun that was used. Aaron told his colleagues that they needed to bring this person in for questioning. Not only did they arrest him, but they found the gun on him as well. The homicide was solved. In addition, the detectives connected the gun to other shooting incidents in the city thanks to a close look at the ballistic reports. That's retroactive policing at its most effective. This particular case is also a strong example of what being respectful and decent as a beat cop can do for you down the line. Aaron was smart enough to know that his strategic, proactive actions meant something. This is a singular example, though. What about an entire city? Coming off an awful couple of years, Minneapolis made some concessions in how they address public safety, without going the full defund route.

In 2022, the city launched Operation Endeavor, a program that uses data to find the areas where crime is having the most impact so that the city can funnel resources to those areas—not just resources for law enforcement but also for violence prevention, outreach, and peace groups. They don't want to just arrest people in these areas; they want to actually engage them. This operation is partly a response to the declining number of officers in the department, but the results speak for themselves. During the first month of the operation, from late September to late October 2022, the number of gunshot wound victims and calls reporting gun crimes went down by nearly 30 percent each, compared with the same time period in 2021. It's a small sample size and it'll take time to see what its long-term effects are, but the strategy on the part of the police and the city as a whole should be encouraging. "Better does not mean good," Minneapolis mayor Jacob Frey said at a press conference about the operation. "The fact that things are improving substantially based on the data does not mean we are where we want to be. We are keeping our nose to the grindstone. We will continue to review the data and make sure we are deploying the resources to where they are most effective."

The police in Buffalo, New York, took similar actions. In 2022, the city employed the hot-spot policing method after back-to-back years of nearly record homicides and shootings. But the cops aren't just racking up low-level arrests in the areas that struggle with violence. They're engaging respectfully with people in these spots, using data-driven intel and investigative techniques. It's all evidence-based work. Guess what? It's leading to positive results. Halfway through 2022, Buffalo had a 36 percent decrease in shootings compared with 2021. "This new strategy, which is very data-driven, where we identify hot spots and then send police into hot spots for foot patrol has helped to build the community and police relationship," Buffalo mayor Byron Brown previously said. They're not focused on everyday citizens, they're focused on those committing violent crimes and the ones who they know have done it before. These same kinds of actions have been taken in other cities. There's proof that proactive and retroactive investigations are effective. Imagine how much more of this work the police would be able to do well if they didn't focus on the issues they're not equipped to handle.

For example, in Eugene, Oregon, mobile crisis workers and medical professionals have routinely been responding to certain public safety, mental health, and medical calls rather than the police for nearly three decades. Because the small city has decided to fully invest in a program that employs well-trained social workers and other medical professionals, they're able to operate fully while the police focus on the problems they're trained to deal with. Residents in the city know that they can call CAHOOTS, which is the nonprofit mobile crisis intervention program that Eugene uses, and not have to worry about a police officer showing up with a gun. This fits into the overall strategy for addressing gun violence.

Boston has been an unsung exemplar for addressing firearm violence the right way. It's one of the 30 largest cities in the country, but it has some of the lowest shooting and homicide numbers. It is the same size as Las Vegas; Portland, Oregon; Louisville, Kentucky; and Nashville, all of which have much higher numbers. What is Boston doing right? The state and the city have strong gun laws, but its success is also a result of the work of community-based organizations and strong prevention strategies from the police department. Boston is taking a "both-and" approach, rather than the either-or strategy many try to use to address the problem. Shootings are still disproportionately affecting Black people in the city, but the overall numbers show that they're in a much better place than comparable cities. It even does a better job collecting data than other cities. Rather than just have stats on the crimes, the Boston Police Department collects demographic information on crime victims, something experts have begged cities to do a better job of.

There are other cities that are taking effective steps to address gun violence. Dallas mayor Eric Johnson uses strategic hot-spot policing and other evidence-based community prevention efforts to get a handle on crime in his city. And Newark—which historically struggled with crime, violence, and a brutal police department—has done a 180 over the last decade. The city remodeled its approach to public safety to include more collaboration between grassroots organizations and the police. Newark was one of the only cities that didn't see a significant surge in gun violence in 2020. During the social unrest that came after the murder of George Floyd, the protests in Newark were mostly peaceful.

These are cities, communities, and people who are using the very solutions that will have the most impact on addressing gun violence. The long-term investments will take years to really show results—not the investment in better policing and better community-led programs, but the overall investment in the neighborhoods that struggle to thrive. It'll take a lot of pressure and accountability for the local and federal governments to actually put the proper funds and resources into the hood for people to be able to live. But there's too much evidence that shows that when living and community conditions are strong and healthy, crime is less of an issue. This same principle can work for inner-city neighborhoods. Community members need to keep the pressure on their city and state leaders, and city and state leaders need to keep that same pressure on the federal government. Enough experts and community leaders have made it clear that this needs to happen for peace to be sustained. The same goes for laws that are put in place. They'll take some time to really show results, but the initiative has to be there. Like the VICTIMS Act that Florida representative Val Demings put together in 2022. The law would create a grant program within the Department of Justice to help local law enforcement improve their clearance rates for homicides by training officers better and investing in the right technology. It would also provide funding and support—such as resources, housing, and relocation aid—for those on the community side who are gun violence victims or relatives of victims. Demings is a former police chief, but this isn't about giving the police a bunch of money to do whatever they want with it. It's a very specific law with a specific goal that would directly affect the communities where gun violence routinely goes unsolved. It passed in the House in 2022. This wouldn't have an impact right away, but in time, if applied properly, it will.

The same goes for the $26 million in funding that the Department of Justice announced in late 2022. The money will "fund a wide range of research, statistical and evaluation activities." This is the exact type of research funding that experts have been calling for. "Connecting science with policy and practice begins with the most accurate, relevant and timely crime and justice data, and the need for that data has never been greater," the former Bureau of Justice Statistics director Dr. Alexis R. Piquero previously said. "These grants will enable us to collect, compile and disseminate the information our nation's policymakers and practitioners need to make informed decisions about public safety." We can't ignore the nongovernment and non-community-based entities either. Research from experts and criminologists is also vital. Like that of the Center for the Study and Practice of Violence Reduction, which was launched in 2022 by the University of Maryland and crime researcher Thomas Abt. This fully funded research center will focus on addressing community gun violence. "To put it plainly, the mission of the VRC is to save lives by stopping violence," Thomas Abt said at the time the center was launched. "By combining rigorous research with real-world know-how, we can help policymakers make the right choices in this critical public policy area."

Even though it's been difficult to make headway with gun laws, there have been some positive actions taken since 2020. Along with the Bipartisan Safer Communities Act, the governor of Illinois signed a law in 2023 that banned assault weapons and the sale of high-capacity magazines. The Dicky Amendment, which indirectly placed heavy restrictions on federal gun violence research, was amended in 2018. While it's still in place, in 2020 the federal budget included $25 million for the CDC and National Institutes of Health to research gun deaths and injuries. This was the first federal gun violence research funding since 1996. New research will have a tremendous impact in determining best practices for addressing gun violence.

These are examples of actions that were taken in the aftermath of the COVID-19 pandemic, which had put everything to a halt. Remember, before the pandemic, gun violence and homicides nationally were on a downward trend. Some of the worst neighborhoods were becoming safer and safer. There was a bit more harmony in these areas. The country was doing okay in terms of gun violence compared with a couple of years prior, but it wasn't enough to make sure that the systems in place could withstand a global health crisis. And even if the national numbers weren't as bad, there were still certain areas that struggled heavily, like Baltimore. At the same time, some of these proposed solutions weren't at the front of people's minds. Violence intervention and community-based solutions weren't part of the national discussion on gun violence; they were only talked about in certain parts of the criminal justice community.

It's not simply a theory that these suggested solutions can work. They do work. No, they are not perfect. Policing is not perfect, community-led organizations are not perfect, gun laws are not perfect, and efforts to take accountability and responsibility are not perfect. There are going to be failures on all sides. Some of the community violence intervention programs aren't going to work right away, and some of the things the police do aren't going to be celebrated. There is no perfect solution to any complex problem. There are too many variables. That's why the solutions need to be based on evidence, implemented strategically, rigorously analyzed, and adjusted based on new information. That's how they can be truly effective. The circumstances of COVID and other factors upended things, but if these systems had been put in place properly beforehand, then the outside factors would not have been as damaging as they were. The key piece to learn from all of this is that these initiatives can be truly effective if the right effort is put into them.

Just ask those who are actually doing the work.

9

Fight for the Resolution

By the end of the summer of 2022, Roy was cautiously optimistic. There were far fewer shootings in his work area that year. "We've had some incidents but it pales in comparison to previous years," Roy says. As he looks back, there's no doubt in his mind that COVID-19 played a big part in the disruption and chaos that happened. At the same time, if he's being honest with himself, he feels like that time period refocused him and his fellow workers. "It was like a gut check. We had to take a hard look at what we were doing and what we could do in the future if something like this happened again." That's Roy in a nutshell: taking responsibility but understanding that there are other factors outside his control. A change he's noticed on the community side is that people are more accepting of the outreach that he and his team of violence interrupters do. That means a lot to Roy. "I think people are seeing the impact we can have and they appreciate it," he says.

If Roy told you he was 30, you'd believe him, but he's closer to 50, and despite all the time he missed when he was locked up, he's got goals. The first thing is that he needs to be here for his family, and he needs them to feel reassured about his job. They're not naive: they know that his work can be dangerous and put him in deadly situations. "In this line of work, the people that you love have concerns about you being out there and doing this work," he says. But beyond that, he thinks a lot about his legacy. What is he leaving behind? What can he pass on to his children, nieces, and nephews? Interestingly, he's not sure that his violence interruption work will leave a legacy. If you ask people who know him, they'll say he will always be known in Bed-Stuy for how much healing he's enabled. Part of his legacy is the incredible, selfless, and considerate work he's done for his neighborhood.

But Roy wants to leave more behind for those who are coming up after him, something he feels would be more tangible. One of his goals is to create a curriculum for schools, like lesson plans on conflict resolution and violence prevention. "I would want to have a cognitive foundation to it because a lot of these issues that we're dealing with is a mentality that we're seeing manifest through behavior," he says. He thinks his education from the streets to prison to violence interruption would serve him well in creating such a curriculum. Roy can't understand why New York City schools don't have some kind of education program on gun violence, given how much of it many of the students have to deal with. Roy could see how someone might flinch at the idea of discussing gun violence in schools, but his suggestion is to do so not in a sensationalized and fearful way but in an informative way. Keep in mind, many of these kids deal with it in their daily lives, whether it's through close family members, friends, or just the circumstances in their neighborhoods. Roy would want to teach kids how gun violence, poverty, and education are connected.

Roy gets calls from schools asking him and his team to come and help them mediate conflicts. What stands out to him in those instances is that after they're done dealing with a specific incident, the kids have to come back to school the next day, the next week, with the possibility of the beef spilling out into the streets. He thinks schools are a perfect place for kids to really learn about these issues. "Teachers should be trained on how to have those discussions," he says. That's something Roy is focused on. He's not sure when or how it will materialize, but it's one of the things he sees for himself in the future. "I don't know what that looks like. I don't know if it's something that I do in 5 years or 10 years," he says.

Is Roy going to spend the rest of his life fighting gun violence? Probably not. There's an end in sight for him, which is why the legacy part is so important. If he can leave something real behind that addresses the problem, then that'll overpower the mistakes he made as a youth. But Roy doesn't let that define him. He can't. His work over the past decade is what defines him. That's the beauty of his journey. He went from a big part of the problem to a big part of the solution. There's no shame in leaving the violence prevention field. It's hard work and it's not something someone should do indefinitely. Even with that, Roy does envision himself staying involved for a little while longer because he knows how important the problem is. He sees the lives it's harming. "There's still work to do. Even when it gets better, we still have to do the work," Roy says, with determination in his voice.

That's the sad reality. There's no way to sugarcoat it. Gun violence is a problem. It's a serious problem in poor Black communities. All the data, research, and anecdotes make that clear. Even when the numbers became a bit better before 2020, it remained an issue in the hood. As a country, we've decided where it's okay for daily shootings and deaths to happen. Just take a second to think about that. Really think about it. Take a step back from the talking points, the politics, the pro–law enforcement arguments, the pro–police reform arguments, and everything else on the outside that serves as a distraction. Just forget all of that for a moment.

We have accepted that it's okay for certain communities in this country to deal with constant shootings, carnage, and death. If those words don't mean anything, just look at the graph on this page. Look at who the victims of gun violence are. It's easy to see that our country doesn't care about them. Not just one community or a few but entire populations and neighborhoods are allowed to suffer from gunfire and nonstop killings. If a news report came out and it said, "15 people died in the city of Chicago," without any real context, people would be frantic and concerned. But once the news report explained that it was 15 Black people who were killed on the South Side of Chicago, people would check out and feel like it didn't apply to them.

Our government leaders have made it clear that it's okay for a child to be sitting in the backseat of a car and catch a stray bullet. It's okay for students to have to crawl under their desks because a gunman is lurking in the halls of their school. There's no problem with people going to the grocery store or the mall and having to think about where the closest exit is in case someone comes in to shoot up the place. Children today are more likely to die from a gun than they are from a car accident. That's all children. Multiply that four times (yes, four) for Black children. It's okay that most

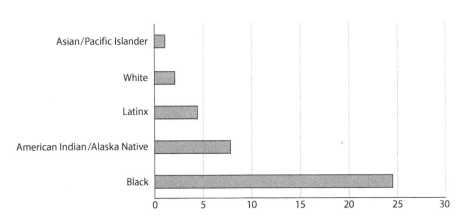

Firearm homicide death rate per 100,000 by race, 2018–2021.
Source: CDC; see https://everystat.org/.

young Black men in America die from gunshot wounds. It's okay for gun violence to be a leading cause of death for Black women too. The same goes for Latino men. It's okay for members of minority groups to get gunned down on a regular basis. That's what our country has said with its actions for over 30 years. Look at what happened to the Black community in the 1970s, '80s, and '90s. Gun violence is just a symptom of the problems that emerged during that time period. Sure, we've gone through periods of relative peace, but it was never sustained.

We can argue for an eternity about why it got worse in 2020. Blame the pandemic and the strain it caused in the country. Blame the antipolice rhetoric and how criminals took advantage of it. Say it's easy to access guns. Blame hip-hop if you want to. Tell people in the hood that it's their fault and that they just need to do better. Get a megaphone and say it's lack of faith that's driving this. We can use election cycles to talk about murders in the hood and why one party has failed while the other party says they know how to address it. But anyone who is really paying attention knows that you can't blame this on one particular factor, and trying to do so is not going to lead to any solutions. The argument should no longer be about what causes this. That's short-sighted, and we're past it.

With all of that said, we can fix this. All the tools that are needed to correct this problem are available in this country. There's no holy grail of solutions that needs to be discovered. We know exactly what works and what doesn't work. We just have to apply the solutions properly. Addressing poverty and socioeconomic issues needs to be a priority for the government. Community-led programs and nonenforcement government programs that tackle gun violence have to work together in some capacity. The police have to be more strategic in their actions.

Community organizations need to use evidence-based tools and methods. The federal government has to find a way to stem the flow of illegal weapons. The community itself has to step up and do its part. In the big picture, that's it. Plain and simple.

These solutions can't be applied on their own. It's not going to work if we only invest in the communities and don't get a handle on the trafficking. Shootings and killings will not drop if we invest in community-led organizations without rigorous research and evaluations. Efforts among residents to take more responsibility for gun violence won't be sustainable on their own if the police target every Black male between 18 and 25 who lives in the hood. This isn't an either-or situation; it's a both-and issue. We can address the long-term systemic issues in the hood while also reducing crime and violence. We've tried the single-solution approach to gun violence before. It didn't work, or rather it wasn't sustainable.

We tried the all-police route, most notably in the 1990s, which had grave consequences. The blame for those consequences doesn't only fall on the shoulders of law enforcement or the government. Crime during that period was a major concern, especially for people in poor Black communities (where it remains a concern today). So the policies that were put in place to take a hyper-police, tough-on-crime approach were celebrated by residents in the hood who just wanted the criminals and guns off the street. Many pro-law enforcement experts and researchers will say it worked. It worked for politicians who wanted to be tough on crime and it worked for police departments that were rewarded for doing the kind of policing that doesn't actually fix anything. The numbers tend to back it up to a point. If you look at New York City, for example, there was a period where violence was down and police arrests, police stops, and incarceration were all going down. That's great, but the communities were still poor, there were still guns flooding the neighborhoods, and people couldn't get good jobs. Policing by itself was only going to work up to a point. Then a once-in-a-lifetime pandemic hit, which was compounded by a tragedy that severely fractured the relationship between police and the community, a relationship that was already tense. Those same pro–law enforcement voices say that the reason gun violence went up is that the country moved away from policing. That's partly true (we've never done strategic policing in a large-scale way), but we never addressed any of the other factors, so the success of law enforcement wasn't going to last, even if every police department in the country focused on violent crime the right way.

This isn't to denigrate the police. They have a very important role to play in all of this. The point here is that one solution isn't going to cut it, and policing is the one solution we've prioritized. What drove the surge in gun violence in 2020 was a combination of factors. The solutions are also going to be a combination of factors. There are those who say that gun violence isn't nearly as bad as it was in the 1990s. Their point is that we shouldn't be making that big a deal about it because "it's not as bad as it used to be." If you look at the overall numbers that's true, but the people who make this point don't realize just how disrespectful it is. It's disrespectful to the victims, the relatives of the victims, the residents, the community leaders, the police, and everyone else who has to deal with this problem on a daily basis. Don't tell Roy that it's not as bad as it was in the 1990s. Don't tell that to people who live in Philadelphia, Baltimore, St. Louis, Minneapolis, Memphis, Kansas City, Louisville, Detroit, and Jackson. The murder rate increase nationally from 2019 to 2020 was the largest single-year increase since the 1960s. Most of those murders happened with a gun, and most of them happened in the hood.

This issue has become political, just like many other serious issues. Politicians love talking about gun violence; they love to bring it up when tragedy strikes. Think of all the press conferences you've seen after a deadly mass shooting. The mayors and governors declare that gun violence needs to stop. They vow to do everything they can to end the pain. But when it's time to sit in their offices with their team and actually do the work it takes to address the epidemic, politics get in the way. They can't just throw money at the hood because that's not an acceptable thing to do as a politician. They can't reward good policing because that takes too much effort and time—it's easier to just be a proponent of simplistic law enforcement strategies. Local politicians certainly don't want to go to war with the gun industry and make gun trafficking in their municipalities a priority. The political party that complains about its opponents being soft on crime is okay with making it easier for people to openly carry the deadliest types of weapons without training or permits. That party is actually the one that's soft on crime when you take into account the number of mass shootings that happen every year with high-capacity assault rifles.

Politics is in the way of fixing this. It shouldn't be. If we took the politics out of it and looked at it like a public health crisis, then we could bypass all the back-and-forth. We can have different opinions on what's driving it, but we need to come together on the solutions. Political leaders need to have the courage to step up and refuse to compromise with the gun lobby when it comes to gun violence. They can no longer shortcut around it. It's too important at the local level. Funding and resources can (and should) come from the federal government, but it's the local leaders, cops, and community members who bear the brunt of the actual implementation. Cities should look at comparable communities that are addressing the problem effectively and learn from them. The same goes for the community side. The stakeholders need to be aware of what works and what doesn't. Pragmatic solutions exist, but we need to let go of the political ideologies that are preventing us from implementing them.

We also need patience. This isn't going to get fixed overnight. If local governments and communities truly come together to tackle gun violence in the long term, it'll take years for things to turn around in a large-scale way. And even after that, the solutions will need to be continually applied. We can't try something for a year or two, not see immediate results, and abandon it. We should be asking, How can it improve? What needs to happen for it to work more effectively? These are the questions to consider instead of simply getting rid of something. Not to bag on the police again, but we've given them over 100 years to get things right and they haven't fixed the problem. Yes, there have been periods when the issue improved as a result of policing, but again, it didn't last. We have to commit to all of the solutions, and we have to commit to them for the long haul. The will to do it must be there, and it must remain there when times are tough or getting better. Gun violence is not going to just disappear, but the country can lessen its impact and address it in a meaningful way.

What happens when another life-altering event takes place in America? What safeguards are going to be in place to make sure this type of problem doesn't surge again? If the country commits to long-term, sustainable solutions, then that event won't have as much of an impact on the problem. Plus, the most disenfranchised and vulnerable communities won't be forced to carry even more weight than they already do. We can't let a lull in the numbers stop us from continuing the work. We need to treat this like it's a persistent problem because it is. There is no perfect solution, and no one who is being serious is advocating for perfection. What they're calling for is a sustainable commitment to addressing the issues.

Everyone has a role to play. Everyone can take action. Even the people who are not directly affected by gun violence. We should not be okay with people getting shot and killed every day in this country. Not when there are solutions to the problem. It's simply about will at this point. Black people in the hood have that will and do the work without any applause or praise. Who else has the will and courage to step up? From the community side to those on the streets, the beat cops, the politicians, the police chiefs, the lawmakers in Congress, the researchers, the advocates, the regular civilians—who among them is going to make a concerted effort for change? If the answer isn't all of them, then we won't see sustained change.

There is real hope. With a consistent and diligent fight, we can defeat the epidemic of gun violence.

Epilogue

The Path

"So the concern now is you being in the book at all." That's me, almost panicking on the phone with Roy. I'm on my living-room couch, sweating, shaking my head, rocking back and forth, and thinking, *This can't be happening.* By now, I had done maybe 20 interviews with him over five months after he agreed to be the main source in the book. He was genuinely surprised when I approached him about it (I had previously done a piece on him for my job), but he was a no-brainer for me. In the few years that I had been covering this topic, no one else made sense to be the focal point of the book. Roy is the embodiment of everything important about the gun violence issue. But now, less than two weeks before I have to turn in the manuscript, he's getting cold feet.

He doesn't mind talking about his experiences, but his family is concerned. During the process, I decided to send him the portions of the book that would heavily feature him and his story. I don't know now if that was a mistake, but it felt like the right thing to do at the time. I wanted to make sure that the presentation of his stories was completely accurate, but I also wanted to make sure there weren't things in there he didn't want to be told. I figured if he had an issue with anything, it would be something small, a tiny detail or something insignificant that we could take out. All stories in the book about him are directly from him (and corroborated by public records), and I only know them because he told me. I didn't think there would be entire stories that he would want left out. Well, that's what happened. He wanted entire sections taken out of the book. Rather, his family did. They wanted the shoot-out story taken out, the story about him sitting in the police station, and some of the details about his time in prison. They didn't like the way he came across. I couldn't fathom that. Roy is a hero in my eyes; he's the hero in this book. When I reread his sections in full, I see a man who made some terrible mistakes as a teenager, paid the price for those mistakes, came home, and dedicated his life to improving his community. To me, he represents what America is supposed to be about.

But his family wasn't feeling it and I respected that. We reached a compromise: I'd conceal his name and take out the name of the organization he works for. I didn't have to do that. All our conversations were on the record. Any other journalist probably wouldn't have sent him the sections to review. He wouldn't have seen them till the book came out. I could have just kept his identifying information in the book, but my overall goal was to prioritize the voices of the people who deal with this issue on a daily basis. So how could I ignore the concerns of someone like him who risks his life every day to address this issue? I struggled with this for a while, but in the end I think this was the right decision, and I learned a valuable lesson.

When I first decided to write a book about gun violence, I don't think I truly believed it was going to happen as soon as it did. I started working on the proposal for the book in January 2021, the day after New Year's. I had no book publishing connections. My plan was to write the proposal a page at a time for four months, pretty it up, and just start sending it out (there were *a lot* of rejections). I thought to myself, "Well, if by some miracle I actually get a book deal, it's gonna take a while." Fast-forward to October 2021 and I'm having real conversations with Johns Hopkins University Press about the proposal. In January 2022, they offered me a contract.

I was excited. Me writing a book? The same kid whose mom had to tape-record him in middle school to make sure he was actually reading for his book reports? It didn't feel like real life. But that quickly changed to, "Damn, all the stuff I said I was going to do in that proposal I have to actually do now." So I got to work. I was already reporting on gun violence for my job, but the book brought it to a different level. I contacted over 400 people—police, politicians, community leaders, residents, street-savvy residents, activists, surviving victims, relatives of victims, former cops, former politicians, former ATF directors, experts, researchers, criminologists, gang members, former gang members, drug dealers. I was fortunate enough to travel as well and hear from those same kinds of people in other parts of the country. I wanted to hear from anyone who had experience with gun violence. Anyone who could provide some insight into the solutions. That was the key here. We all know gun violence is a problem, and we all certainly knew by the end of 2020 that gun violence was surging. But I wanted this book to be about solutions. The real solutions, not the hypothetical ones. The ones that we know can work.

That was the focus of all my conversations. What are the solutions to the problem? What needs to happen? What are we not doing well? What are we doing well? The public at large doesn't think about solutions to these kinds of issues. I heard a lot of different answers, but there was also some consistency in what people thought. One thing I learned was how comprehensive the solutions to gun violence need to be. Even when I started covering it for *Time*, I didn't think about it that way. I know most people don't think of it that way. They think it's simple. "The police need to just arrest more people," or "If everyone just puts the gun down this issue would go away." It's actually more complicated than that, and to hear the people I spoke with acknowledge this was surprising. I think in the wake of everything that happened in 2020, we reassessed how we view gun violence and public safety. Not just the public but lawmakers and police as well. I was shocked when police chiefs and detectives were talking about other factors outside of law enforcement. I don't think you'd hear that from them as much before 2020. It's unfortunate that it took such a horrible year for people to shift how they viewed this issue, but that's how it goes sometimes.

Reporting on this was stressful. Not just because it's a difficult and heartbreaking topic but because of how much I learned and how much I wanted everyone else to understand too. One of the more frustrating parts was seeing all the ignorant and uninformed things people would say about gun violence, especially on social media. I'm not just talking about random trolls—I'm talking about criminal justice professors and experts who are supposed to be, well, experts. About a week before the 2022 midterm elections, I was about three chapters away from completing the first draft of the manuscript, so I was at my desk writing.

Okay, I was procrastinating, so I was scrolling through Twitter. What caught my attention at this moment was the discussion about crime and gun violence. Crime is always a hot-button issue around election time. I find it interesting because the crime in the hood (really any issue in the hood) becomes a concern when it's time to vote, but then it's relegated to the back of people's minds in nonelection years. I follow a lot of criminal justice experts, cops, former cops, reporters, and academics on Twitter. For some reason, this evening, the discussion about crime and gun violence drove me crazy.

Is it because I was in the middle of writing this book? Probably. I noticed that I became more aware of posts about the subject. I wanted to respond to every single tweet I saw from a verified account that I thought was wrong-headed or inaccurate. One guy wrongly says, "Gun violence didn't go up at the start of the pandemic, it only went up after George Floyd was killed." Do I waste my time responding to him and say I spoke with over 100 people (law enforcement included) who said gun violence started to get worse shortly after the pandemic began, weeks before George Floyd was killed?

An academic makes the assertion that poverty has nothing to do with gun violence. I want to tell him to go to the corner of Rockaway and Livonia in Brownsville, Brooklyn, and say that over a megaphone (he shouldn't do that: he'd probably get robbed). After pondering and even drafting out responses, I reached what I believe is a logical conclusion: Twitter is not the place to have a real debate about issues like this. As much as I want to say something to people, it's just not worth it to do it over social media. Instead, this book is my response to those people. I'm not the foremost expert on gun violence. Not even close. My hope is that this book will open people's eyes to what a surge in gun violence looks like and what really needs to happen to address it. I've essentially compiled the perspectives of people who have a clue and put them in a book with some stories mixed in. I want the conversation to shift from what's causing the problem to how we can apply the solutions so it's no longer a problem. The big takeaway I hope people grasp is that there is no one solution to gun violence. People need to accept that.

I don't often share my opinions on serious issues publicly. I have a bit of an old-school mentality: I think as a member of the media (which I am), you gotta earn that right. You gotta put in some work for your opinion to have weight. Social media has made it seem like everyone's opinion matters. Trust me, they don't matter much. There wasn't one person I spoke with in the hood who gave a damn about what the internet "experts" or "activists" have to say on Twitter. Y'all are just arguing with each other. But the end of this book feels like the proper place to express some of my opinions.

I think this problem is one of the most pressing ones our country is facing. I don't think we as a country talk about it with enough honesty and sincerity. Our country is more divided than it's ever been in my lifetime. To me, that division doesn't matter when it comes to gun violence. The Left and the Right have fumbled how they handle it. I don't think we collectively care about the problem, because if we truly did, it wouldn't be as bad as it is now. I'm sick of seeing young Black kids killed in their neighborhoods. It hurts my soul. I see my little brother and sister every time I read one of those stories. I don't care about politics. I hate how this issue gets divided along political lines. This is about life and death. Why does it have to be political? If there were one issue that should bypass the political arena, it would be this. I hate that we only seem to come together around gun violence when a high-fatality mass shooting happens in a place that's supposed to be "safe." And even when those happen, we don't do anything about it. I'm sick of hearing politicians say "thoughts and prayers" after a tragic mass shooting. I'm a Christian; I believe in God. Thoughts and prayers don't mean a damn thing without action. But also there are mass shootings in Baltimore and Chicago every weekend. So what if it was on a corner in the hood? People still got shot. America accepts shootings in poor Black neighborhoods. Our country is okay with Black kids getting killed. We're okay with random mass shootings. It makes me sick.

By the time this book comes out, I expect the numbers will be going down and people won't be thinking about this much (unless one of those mass shootings is in the news). Through the first half of 2023, gun violence was steadily declining from the previous year. I expect shootings and murders nationally will still be higher than pre-pandemic levels, but because the country will have seen a couple of years with decreasing numbers, everyone will think the problem is taking care of itself. While you're thinking that, people in poor neighborhoods are still going to be struggling to tackle gun violence. Unless we're committed to changing it in a meaningful way, the hood is always going to struggle with gun violence. Anyone who reads this book needs to understand that.

Feel free to disagree with the points made in this book, challenge them, or ridicule them. I welcome it. I'm just one person. I wish I could have spoken with thousands of people about this. I had to make do with the ones who were kind enough to spare their time, some of the strongest, most gracious people I've ever come across. That's the last piece of this for me: We've heard enough from those on the outside who have so much to say about gun violence but don't do anything about it. It's time to hear from those who live with this reality.

ACKNOWLEDGMENTS

I'm going to do my best to keep this short, but I have so many people to thank. I think it makes sense to start with the people who directly made this book possible and then move on to the more abstract gratitude. I want to say thank you to all the people who spoke with me. I did over 300 interviews, so I can't list every single one of them, but each one of you brought so much to this book. I'm not an expert on this topic. It's the people I spoke with who deserve the credit for enlightening me and helping me understand the information so I could relay it. It was difficult to get certain people to talk, but I value the perspective of everyone I was able to speak with. Even the ones I had to chase down. You made this book possible.

Roy Alfonso opened up in a way that I don't think he expected to. He told me stories that he'd never told anyone before. I don't want to take credit for that; I think our interviews became cathartic for him, and I also think he felt compelled to share his experiences around the issue. Whatever the case is, I'm indebted to him. The book doesn't work without him. I hope his story inspires others the way it inspired me. I hope he sees himself the way I see him when he reads this.

To the people I spoke with who lost loved ones and friends to gun violence, I want to again offer my deepest condolences and thank you for sparing the time you did with me. To those I spoke with who were victims of gun violence, thank you for allowing me to ask you questions and hear your stories. Each and every one of you had an irrefutable strength about you. Thank you for allowing me to share your thoughts and perspectives on this critical issue. Yours were the voices I set out to prioritize in this book, and I hope I've done that.

To all the community leaders and activists I spoke with, thank you for sharing your expertise with me. You all put the issue in the proper context and I am thankful for that. I'm also grateful to the everyday residents I spoke with on the streets, in their homes, and at community board meetings, among other places. These are the folks who sometimes get ignored in the coverage of gun violence: the people who have to live in the communities that are plagued by it.

I also want to thank those in law enforcement who spoke with me, both past and present members. There's a lot of scrutiny aimed at police officers in this country, and they've certainly earned that, but there are high-character, decent people working in police departments who truly care about gun violence. Just like community workers who are on the ground trying to fix this, police officers are doing the same.

I'm grateful as well to the experts who study the data and crunch all the numbers. You all have a perspective that I never could, and while I'm critical of some of these experts and their bird's-eye view, we need that perspective to address this issue. I also want to give a specific thank-you to David Simon, creator of *The Wire*, who is one of my idols. Interviewing and quoting him in my first book is wild!

Thank you to Johns Hopkins University Press for believing in the idea for this book and providing the resources necessary to complete it. To my editor, Robin Coleman, I can't thank you enough. I'm not sure I could have been matched with a better editor for my first book. You made the process easier and less daunting. Your notes and edits helped me take a step back when I was too deep in the weeds. You made yourself available when I ran into issues. Every author should have the opportunity to work with an editor like you.

Okay, now I'm moving over to the people who had a more indirect role in this. Grace Shadid, your name is nowhere else in this book, but I wouldn't have finished it without you by my side. You were there from the moment I started working on the proposal. You let me bounce ideas off you, you were my first call when I ran into roadblocks, you let me vent, and you read portions before anyone else did. You stayed on the phone with me for hours at a time when I struggled. I think there were moments when you believed in this book more than I did. I'm so blessed to have you in my life.

I have to thank my family—all of you, not just the ones who spoke with me for the preface. You all give me strength, and you're all the reason I'm able to do this work. It's the laughs and the time spent with you that I think about when I'm sitting at my desk struggling to write. I love all of you. To my parents, Desiree McDougald and Neville Bates, I hope you guys know how grateful I am for all that you've done and continue to do. A special thank-you to David Mogle and his dad for helping me on my reporting trip to Youngstown. We're brothers for life!

To the great editors and mentors I've had: Lily Rothman, Michael Zennie, Tina Susman, Christy Oglesby, Calvin Lawrence Jr., Wil Cruz, Blake Morrison, Simone Weichselbaum, and Mensah Dean. I'm a better writer because of all of you. To the reporters I've had the privilege to work with: Karl Vick, Andrew Chow, Jasmine Aguilera, Janell Ross, Maddie Carlisle, Charlotte Alter, and Armando Garcia. I appreciate all I learned from working with each of you.

I have to give special shout-outs to Alex Rees and Tami Luhby, who are more than editors, mentors, and colleagues. These are two people I revere. They're two of the best journalists in the business. Everything I've learned from them helped me craft this book.

Petty sidenote here, but to the leaders of Grace Church School, specifically George Davidson, thank you for kicking me out of middle school. Y'all didn't know the fuel you'd give me for the rest of my life and how that fuel would help me in my toughest moments when writing this book. I'm glad I get to prove y'all wrong for as long as I live. You didn't know God was on my side.

And lastly, I want to thank everyone who read this book. I hope you've learned more about this issue and how urgent it is that we address it.

ESSAY ON SOURCES

There's a lot of information and reporting in this book, and I'm sure readers are interested in where it came from. I can start by saying that many of the quotes you see are from interviews I did myself, but the statistics, the data, and some of the other information come from a variety of sources, which are listed here.

As mentioned in the preface, a few of my interlocutors' names are pseudonyms. If you read the epilogue, you know Roy is one of them. The others are Bobby, Tion, Kellen, Todd Morris, Sharod, and Detective Aaron Clayton. These are the folks who were happy to talk but didn't want their names in the book.

The data on the annual costs of gun violence in the United States cited in the preface are derived from a July 2022 report by Everytown for Gun Safety: "The Economic Cost of Gun Violence," Everytown Research and Policy, July 19, 2022, https://everytownresearch.org /report/the-economic-cost-of-gun-violence/.

In chapter 1, the data on New York City's crime and incarceration rates are from a tweet Vital City posted: Vital City (@VitalCityNYC), "From 2017 to 2019, the city's crime and incarceration rates were at an all-time low. This was a remarkable achievement. Many remember the early '90s in the city . . . ," Twitter, December 16, 2022, https:// twitter.com/VitalCityNYC/status/1603784774002393090. Information about Tyler Malden's previous run-ins with the law can be found in Katie Smith, "Police Arrest 2 Chicago Men in Connection with Johnsburg Car Burglary, Fleeing," *Northwest Herald*, September 28, 2018, https://www.shawlocal.com/2018/09/27/police-arrest -2-chicago-men-in-connection-with-johnsburg-car-burglary-fleeing /an7um3p/. The quote from Erikka Gordon appeared in an ABC7 Chicago piece: Craig Wall and Diane Pathieu, "Chicago Shootings: 64

Shot, 11 Fatally in Weekend Violence," ABC7 Eyewitness News, July 13, 2020, https://abc7chicago.com/chicago-shooting-shootings-this -weekend-violence-how-many-shot-in/6314582/. The quote from Taren Weaver, Darius Lee's mother, is from an *Amsterdam News* article: Tandy Lau, Mal'akiy 17 Allah, and Nayaba Arinde, "'He Was Perfect,' Says Kin of Slain Harlem Native Darius Lee, Super Scholar & Rising College Basketball Star," *New York Amsterdam News,* June 23, 2022, https://amsterdamnews.com/news/2022/06/23/he-was-perfect -says-kin-of-slain-harlem-native-darius-lee-super-scholar-rising -college-basketball-star/. When I talk about how Black Americans are disproportionately affected by gun violence, much of that information comes from the Centers for Disease Control and Prevention: Thomas R. Simon et al., "Notes from the Field: Increases in Firearm Homicide and Suicide Rates—United States, 2020–2021," *Morbidity and Mortality Weekly Report* 71, no. 40 (October 7, 2022): 1286–1287, http://dx.doi.org/10.15585/mmwr.mm7140a4. Data for 2018 and 2019 by the Education Fund to Stop Gun Violence, which uses CDC data, are from https://efsgv.org/report/gun-violence-in -america-2018-data-brief-january-2020/. If you want to get more specific, you can look at police data from different cities, which should show the racial breakdown of homicide victims and how they were killed. FBI data will show that gun deaths rose in almost every major city in 2020. The Gun Violence Archive quote is from "General Methodology," Gun Violence Archive, last updated May 31, 2023, https:// www.gunviolencearchive.org/methodology; and the data from the archive were taken from "Past Summary Ledgers," Gun Violence Archive, August 3, 2023, https://www.gunviolencearchive.org/past-tolls. The Council on Criminal Justice data are from "Impact Report: COVID-19 and Crime," Council on Criminal Justice, January 31, 2021, https://counciloncj.org/impact-report-covid-19-and-crime-6/; and the quote is from "About Us," Council on Criminal Justice, accessed August 3, 2023, https://counciloncj.org/ccj-about-us/. The information on racial disparities in gun violence in Washington, DC, is from a National Institute for Criminal Justice Reform report, *Gun Violence Problem Analysis Summary Report: Washington, D.C.* (December 2021), https://cjcc.dc.gov/sites/default/files/dc/sites/cjcc/release_content

/attachments/DC%20Gun%20Violence%20Problem%20Analy
sis%20Summary%20Report.pdf. The data for New York City were
compiled from "Crime and Enforcement Activity Reports," NYPD, accessed August 3, 2023, https://www.nyc.gov/site/nypd/stats/reports
-analysis/crime-enf.page.

CDC data on firearms as the leading cause of death for children and
teenagers in 2020 were taken from https://www.nejm.org/doi/full/10
.1056/NEJMc2201761.

Data on police killings is tricky. The most reliable information only
goes back to the early 2010s. For the stat in chapter 1 on police killing
1,000 people a year, I used Mapping Police Violence, which collects
information from local and state agencies and publicly available media reports: "Mapping Police Violence," Campaign Zero, last updated
June 15, 2023, https://mappingpoliceviolence.org/. Data on firearm
homicide rates by state are from "Firearm Mortality by State," CDC,
last updated March 1, 2022, https://www.cdc.gov/nchs/pressroom
/sosmap/firearm_mortality/firearm.htm. The 28 percent increase
in gun deaths in rural areas in 2020 is from the CDC, https://mis
souriindependent.com/2022/11/17/rural-gun-deaths-exceed-urban
-rates-by-28-because-of-increased-suicide-rates/#:~:text=In%20
2020%2C%20the%20rural%20gun,America%2C%20according
%20to%20CDC%20reports. The murder rates for New York City are
from "Factsheet: 2020 Shootings & Murders," NYC Mayor's Office
of Criminal Justice, January 29, 2021, https://criminaljustice.city
ofnewyork.us/wp-content/uploads/2021/01/2020-Shootings-and
-Murder-factsheet_January-2021.pdf. The discussion on the increased
lethality of gun violence is based on Deidre McPhillips, "Gun Violence in the US Has Become More Lethal, Research Suggests," CNN,
April 5, 2023, https://www.cnn.com/2023/04/05/health/gun-violence
-more-lethal.

In chapter 2, the historical information on inequalities in the poverty rate is from John Creamer, "Inequalities Persist Despite Decline
in Poverty for All Major Race and Hispanic Origin Groups," US Cen-
sus Bureau, September 15, 2020, https://www.census.gov/library
/stories/2020/09/poverty-rates-for-blacks-and-hispanics-reached
-historic-lows-in-2019.html. The quotes from Marvin Bradley and

Teresa Bradley are from *New York Times* articles: Richard A. Oppel Jr. et al., "The Fullest Look Yet at the Racial Inequity of Coronavirus," *New York Times*, July 5, 2020, https://www.nytimes.com/interactive /2020/07/05/us/coronavirus-latinos-african-americans-cdc-data .html; and David Leonhardt, "Covid and Race," *New York Times*, June 9, 2022, https://www.nytimes.com/2022/06/09/briefing/covid -race-deaths-america.html. The quote from Rodney Phillips about Chicagoans dealing with gun violence and the coronavirus at the same is from a *Time* article that I wrote: Josiah Bates, "'We're Catching It Double.' Amid Coronavirus Lockdowns, Gun Violence Continues to Plague Chicago," *Time*, April 11, 2020, https://time.com/5818553/gun -violence-chicago-coronavirus/. The Corey Brooks quote is from that same article. The quote from Dr. Dorian Alexander is from a CNN article: Mark Morales, "A Hospital Slammed by Covid-19 in Spring Sees a New Wave of Patients in Summer—Gunshot Victims," CNN, September 5, 2020, https://www.cnn.com/2020/09/05/us/nyc-hospital -gun-violence/index.html. The information on total gun purchases is from "U.S. Firearms Sales December 2020: Sales Increases Slowing Down, Year's Total Sales Clock in at 23 Million Units," Small Arms Analytics, January 5, 2021, http://smallarmsanalytics.com/v1/pr/2021 -01-05.pdf. The information on first-time gun buyers is from "NSSF Retailer Surveys Indicate 5.4 Million First-Time Gun Buyers in 2021," NSSF, January 25, 2022, https://www.nssf.org/articles/nssf-retailer -surveys-indicate-5-4-million-first-time-gun-buyers-in-2021/. The discussion about the increase in the use of guns in crimes is based on Jeff Asher and Rob Arthur, "The Data Are Pointing to One Major Driver of America's Murder Spike," *Atlantic*, January 10, 2022, https:// www.theatlantic.com/ideas/archive/2022/01/gun-sales-murder -spike/621196/. The Trace article consulted is Champe Barton, "New Data Suggests a Connection between Pandemic Gun Sales and Increased Violence," Trace, December 8, 2021, https://www.thetrace .org/2021/12/atf-time-to-crime-gun-data-shooting-pandemic/. The information on domestic violence shootings is from Dan Glun, "A Handful of States Fueled a National Increase in Domestic Violence Shooting Deaths as COVID-19 Spread," Frontline, June 2, 2021, https://www.pbs.org/wgbh/frontline/article/national-increase

-domestic-violence-shooting-deaths-during-covid-19/. The data on COVID-19's effect in Los Angeles in 2020 can be found in Associated Press, "Density, Poverty Keep Los Angeles Struggling against Virus," *Latino USA*, May 26, 2020, https://www.latinousa.org/2020/05/26 /densitypovertyla/. The number of gun crimes in Grand Rapids in 2020 is from Luke Laster, "GRPD Presents 2020 Crime Report to City Committee," Wood TV, July 27, 2021, https://www.woodtv.com/news /grand-rapids/grpd-presents-2020-crime-report-to-city-committee/. The number of homicides is from John Agar, "Grand Rapids' Killings Hit High in 2020: 'Nobody Deserves to Be Hurt like This,'" MLive, January 1, 2021, https://www.mlive.com/news/grand-rapids/2021/01 /grand-rapids-killings-hit-high-in-2020-nobody-deserves-to-be -hurt-like-this.html.

More information about ShotSpotter, which is mentioned in chapter 3, can be found here: "ShotSpotter Frequently Asked Questions," SoundThinking, accessed August 4, 2023, https://www.soundthinking .com/faqs/shotspotter-faqs/. The quote from Motique Graves is from a *New York Daily News* article: Kerry Burke and Rocco Parascandola, "'Drop the Gun!' Cops Yelled to a Brooklyn Man. He Didn't, and Died in a 62-Bullet Fusillade, Body Camera Footage Shows," *New York Daily News*, July 31, 2020, https://www.nydailynews.com/new-york/nyc -crime/ny-bwc-footage-brooklyn-shooting-nypd-suspect-62-shots -20200731-zvkxiirprbhprdtsdlpyw2bmdq-story.html. The information about the peacefulness of the 2020 protests against the police is from Sanya Mansoor, "93% of Black Lives Matter Protests Have Been Peaceful, New Report Finds," *Time*, September 5, 2020, https://time.com /5886348/report-peaceful-protests/. The discussion of the fear and uneasiness felt by Black people in confrontations with the police is based on Corey Williams and Aaron Morrison, "Police Stops of Black People Often Filled with Fear, Anxiety," AP, April 16, 2022, https:// apnews.com/article/patrick-lyoya-grand-rapids-michigan-george -floyd-8076c7901602d04ddbfdee3d1d352b9c. I also mention how Black men are usually viewed as a threat by the public. You can read more about that in a study published by the American Psychological Association: John Paul Wilson, Kurt Hugenberg, and Nicholas O. Rule, "Racial Bias in Judgments of Physical Size and Formidability: From

Size to Threat," *Journal of Personality and Social Psychology* 113, no. 1 (2017): 59–80, https://www.apa.org/pubs/journals/releases/psp -pspi0000092.pdf. The $1 billion number for the cost of the damages from the 2020 protests and riots came from the Insurance Information Institute, which gathers national insurance claim data: Jennifer A. Kingson, "Exclusive: $1 Billion-Plus Riot Damage Is Most Expensive in Insurance History," Axios, September 16, 2020, https://www.axios .com/2020/09/16/riots-cost-property-damage. I discuss the response of voters to the 2021 ballot question on replacing the police with a department of public safety in Minneapolis in an article I wrote for *Time*: Josiah Bates, "In Blow to 'Defund' Movement, Minneapolis Residents Vote against Replacing the City's Police Department," *Time*, November 3, 2021, https://time.com/6112977/minneapolis-election-defund -police-vote/. Information on the fiscal budget for the New York Police Department can be found in Council of the City of New York, *Report to the Committees on Finance and Public Safety on the Fiscal 2022 Executive Budget for the New York Police Department* (New York: Finance Division, Council of the City of New York, 2021), https:// council.nyc.gov/budget/wp-content/uploads/sites/54/2021/05 /NYPD.pdf. Data on nationwide police funding can be found in "Police Funding Increased Nationwide in 2022: Analysis," Crime Report, October 17, 2022, https://thecrimereport.org/2022/10/17/police -funding-increased-nationwide-in-2022/. The information on the costs incurred from police brutality cases in Milwaukee is from "12 News Investigates: Milwaukee Paid $40M+ in Police Brutality Cases," WISN 12 News, November 10, 2020, https://www.wisn.com/article/12 -news-investigates-milwaukee-paid-dollar40m-in-police-brutality -cases/34618638. The number for Chicago's police misconduct cases is from Chuck Goudie et al., "Chicago Has Authorized Nearly $67M in Police Misconduct Settlement Payments So Far This Year," ABC 7 Eyewitness News, December 13, 2021, https://abc7chicago.com /chicago-police-department-misconduct-payout/11336008/; and the one for New York City is from Samantha Max, "NYPD Lawsuit Payouts on Track to Be Highest in Recent History," Gothamist, August 4, 2022, https://gothamist.com/news/nypd-lawsuit-payouts-on-track-to -be-highest-in-recent-history. The Gallup poll on Black Americans' desire to have policing in their neighborhoods is discussed in Jocelyn Grzeszczak, "81% of Black Americans Don't Want Less Police Presence Despite Protests—Some Want More Cops: Poll," *Newsweek*, August 5, 2020, https://www.newsweek.com/81-black-americans-dont-want-less-police-presence-despite-protestssome-want-more-cops-poll-1523093. The Pew article that lists violence and crime as the number one concern for Black adults is Kiana Cox and Christine Tamir, "Place and Community," Pew Research Center, April 14, 2022, https://www.pewresearch.org/race-ethnicity/2022/04/14/black-americans-place-and-community/. The quote from Nekima Levy Armstrong is from a *Time* article I worked on with a colleague: Josiah Bates and Lissandra Villa, "'You Can Only Demean People So Much.' Minneapolis Activists Aren't Surprised a National Movement Started There," *Time*, June 3, 2020, https://time.com/5846248/minneapolis-george-floyd-police-activists/.

The reference in chapter 4 to East New York as the city's killing fields is from Ashley Southall, "Once the 'Killing Fields,' East New York Has No Murders in 2018," *New York Times*, April 20, 2018, https://www.nytimes.com/2018/04/20/nyregion/east-new-york-precinct-no-murders.html. I go into great detail on the federal investigation into the Louisville Police Department and their handling of the Breonna Taylor case. There are plenty of public Department of Justice statements and news reports that explain the charges against officers in the Place-Based Investigations Unit. The information on Operation Ceasefire is from "Kennedy Trying 'Ceasefire' Again in Baltimore, Site of Earlier 'Disaster,'" Crime Report, February 18, 2014, https://thecrimereport.org/2014/02/18/2014-02-d-kennedy-return-to-baltimore/. The quotes from David Kennedy about Ceasefire are from a Minnesota Public Radio interview: "Bright Ideas with David Kennedy," MPR News, October 25, 2011, https://www.mprnews.org/story/2011/10/25/bright-ideas-david-kennedy. The percentage of people who are locked up for violent crimes is from Wendy Sawyer and Peter Wagner, "Mass Incarceration: The Whole Pie 2023," Prison Policy Initiative, March 14, 2023, https://www.prisonpolicy.org/reports/pie2023.html. The decline in murders in Chicago in 2018 is discussed in "561 Murdered in Chicago in 2018, Down from 660 in 2017," ABC7

Eyewitness News, January 1, 2019, https://abc7chicago.com/chicago
-crime-stats-2018-murders/4999908/. Information on the historical
pattern of police discrimination in Minneapolis can be found in "MN
Human Rights Probe Finds Pattern of Racism in Minneapolis Police
Department," MPR News, April 27, 2022, https://www.mprnews.org
/story/2022/04/26/george-floyd-killing-minnesota-human-rights
-investigation.

In chapter 5 I talk about promising data on the impact of Cure Violence. If you go to their website, you'll find independent studies done
on different Cure Violence sites across the country and the world. Also
see Cure Violence, *The Evidence of Effectiveness* (Chicago: Cure Violence, 2022), https://cvg.org/wp-content/uploads/2022/09/Cure
-Violence-Evidence-Summary.pdf. More information about READI
Chicago can be found in "READI," UChicago Crime Lab, accessed
August 7, 2023, https://urbanlabs.uchicago.edu/programs/readi. The
quote from Rick Rosenfeld about his Cure Violence analysis in
St. Louis is from a *Time* article I wrote: Josiah Bates, "A New Study
Casts Doubt on One of the Country's Most Popular Violence Prevention Approaches," *Time*, February 23, 2022, https://time.com/6148886
/cure-violence-st-louis-effectiveness/. The John Jay College analysis
of violence outreach can be found in "Reducing Violence without
Police: A Review of Research Evidence," John Jay College of Criminal Justice, November 9, 2020, https://johnjayrec.nyc/2020/11/09
/av2020/. Information on the 2015 study of the Pittsburgh program is
from Jeffrey A. Butts et al., "Cure Violence: A Public Health Model to
Reduce Gun Violence," *Annual Review of Public Health* 36 (2015): 39–
53, https://doi.org/10.1146/annurev-publhealth-031914-122509. The
2022 study of READI Chicago is discussed in Andy Grimm, "Arrests,
Shootings Plunged among Those Who Took Part in Anti-violence Program, Even as Crime Spiked in City, New Study Finds," *Chicago Sun-
Times*, April 21, 2022, https://chicago.suntimes.com/crime/2022/4/21
/23004981/readi-chicago-anti-violence-gun-university-uchicago.
The Tyshawn Lee case is covered in Josiah Bates, "Two Chicago Men
Found Guilty of the 'Targeted Execution' of 9-Year-Old Tyshawn Lee.
Here's What to Know about the Crime, and Their Trial," *Time*, last
updated October 4, 2019, https://time.com/5680614/tyshawn-lee

-shooting-chicago-gun-murder-trial/. The quote from Linda Rogers Fulton is in "Natalia Wallace, 7-Year-Old Fatally Shot July 4th, Was 'Sweet, Shy, Loving, and Good at Math,' Family Says," CBS News Chicago, July 5, 2020, https://www.cbsnews.com/chicago/news/natalia -wallace-shot-and-killed-chicago-south-austin/. More information about the underfunding of the court system can be found in "TIPS Toolkit for Fair Court Funding," American Bar Association, June 1, 2016, https://www.americanbar.org/groups/tort_trial_insurance _practice/court_funding1/. President Joe Biden's Build Back Better Framework is presented in "The Build Back Better Framework," White House, accessed August 7, 2023, https://www.whitehouse.gov/build -back-better/. The quote from the White House's statement on its investment in community violence intervention programs is from "Fact Sheet: Biden-Harris Administration Announces Initial Actions to Address the Gun Violence Public Health Epidemic," White House, April 7, 2021, https://www.whitehouse.gov/briefing-room/statements -releases/2021/04/07/fact-sheet-biden-harris-administration -announces-initial-actions-to-address-the-gun-violence-public-health -epidemic/. The text of the Bipartisan Safer Communities Act can be found here: "Bipartisan Safer Communities Act," website of Senator Chris Murphy, accessed August 7, 2023, https://www.murphy.senate .gov/imo/media/doc/bipartisan_safer_communities_act_one_pager .pdf. The Chris Murphy quote is from a tweet he posted on June 21, 2022: Chris Murphy (@ChrisMurphyCT), "Here it is, folks—the Bipartisan Safer Communities Act, the most significant piece of anti-gun violence legislation in nearly 30 years. This bill is going to . . . ," Twitter, June 21, 2022, https://twitter.com/ChrisMurphyCT/status /1539380315201933314. Information on the various grant programs I mention can be found in these sources: "Grant Programs: ONDCP," Office of National Drug Control Policy, accessed August 7, 2023, https://www.whitehouse.gov/ondcp/grant-programs/; "HUD Announces 24 Programs to Join Biden-Harris Administration Justice40 Initiative," US Department of Housing and Urban Development, July 15, 2022, https://www.hud.gov/press/press_releases_media _advisories/hud_no_22_132; "Biden Administration Announces First-Ever Funding Program Dedicated to Reconnecting American

Communities," US Department of Transportation, June 30, 2022, https://www.transportation.gov/briefing-room/biden-administration -announces-first-ever-funding-program-dedicated-reconnecting; Libby Stanford, "Biden Administration Boosts Grants for Community Schools, Sharpens Funding Priorities," *Education Week*, July 12, 2022, https://www.edweek.org/policy-politics/biden-administration -boosts-grants-for-community-schools-sharpens-funding-priorities /2022/07; "Biden Administration Takes Additional Steps to Strengthen Child Nutrition Programs," US Department of Agriculture, June 30, 2022, https://www.fns.usda.gov/news-item/usda-0147.22. The Council on Criminal Justice examines a study of the effect of repairing abandoned houses on gun violence: "Can Repairing Abandoned Housing Reduce Gun Violence?," Council on Criminal Justice, May 19, 2023, https://counciloncj.org/can-repairing-abandoned-housing-reduce -gun-violence/.

A discussion of the data on Black gun ownership, discussed in chapter 6, is in Curtis Bunn, "Why More Black People Are Looking for Safety in Gun Ownership," NBC News, June 14, 2022, https://www .nbcnews.com/news/nbcblk/black-people-are-looking-safety-gun -ownership-rcna32150. The 54 percent increase in guns recovered by police in 2022 is mentioned in Peter Hermann, "D.C. Gun Seizures Are Soaring—but Charges Aren't Sticking," *Washington Post*, June 1, 2022, https://www.washingtonpost.com/dc-md-va/2022/06/01/gun -seizures-dc/; and the comparison data for 2021 is in "2023 Year-to-Date Crime Comparison," Metropolitan Police of Washington, DC, accessed August 7, 2023, https://mpdc.dc.gov/page/district-crime -data-glance. The data are also discussed in Sam Charles and Lourdes Duarte, "A Closer Look at the Chicago Police Department's Gun Recoveries," WGN9 News, https://wgntv.com/news/wgn-investigates/a -closer-look-at-the-chicago-police-departments-gun-recoveries/. The record number of illegal guns seized in New York is covered in "Hochul: Illegal Gun Seizures Up 20% in NY since Launch of Interstate Task Force," NBC New York, August 24, 2022, https://www .nbcnewyork.com/news/local/hochul-ghost-gun-seizures-up-20-in -ny-since-launch-of-interstate-task-force/3837243/#:~:text =Hochul%20also%20announced%20that%20New,the%20history%

200f%20the%20agency. The Giffords Law Center rankings of state gun laws for 2021 can be found in "2021 Annual Gun Law Scorecard," Giffords Law Center, accessed August 7, 2023, https://giffords.org /lawcenter/resources/scorecard2021/. The Everytown for Gun Safety rankings are in "Gun Safety Policies Save Lives," Everytown for Gun Safety, last updated January 12, 2023, https://everytownresearch.org /rankings/. The 1994 assault weapons ban is analyzed in Jeffrey A. Roth and Christopher S. Koper, "Impacts of the 1994 Assault Weapons Ban: 1994–96," National Institute of Justice Research in Brief, March 1999, https://www.ojp.gov/pdffiles1/173405.pdf. The rise of white extremism in the 1990s is traced in Mark Pitcavage, *Surveying the Landscape of the American Far Right* (Washington, DC: George Washington University Program on Extremism, 2019), https://extremism .gwu.edu/sites/g/files/zaxdzs5746/files/Surveying%20The%20 Landscape%20of%20the%20American%20Far%20Right_0.pdf. Gizmodo highlights several government scandals in Lucas Ropek, "10 U.S. Government Scandals You Probably Forgot About," Gizmodo, June 12, 2022, https://gizmodo.com/10-us-government-scandals-you -probably-forgot-about-1849040772. The Steve Dettelbach quote in chapter 6 is from an ABC News interview: "New ATF Director Speaks on His Plans for the Agency," ABC News, July 28, 2022, https://abcnews .go.com/US/atf-director-speaks-plans-agency/story?id=87549962. The decline of the NRA is covered in Giovanni Russonello, "How Much Sway Does the N.R.A. Still Have?," *New York Times*, last updated May 3, 2021, https://www.nytimes.com/2021/04/19/us/politics/nra -gun-control.html. When I say that most Americans support strong gun legislation, that data can be found in many places, including the Pew Research Center, https://www.pewresearch.org/short-reads /2021/09/13/key-facts-about-americans-and-guns/.

In chapter 7, the Bureau of Justice Statistics data on the number of Black people in prison are from E. Ann Carson, *Prisoners in 2020—Statistical Tables* (Washington, DC: US Department of Justice, December 2021), https://bjs.ojp.gov/content/pub/pdf/p20st.pdf. The gender composition can be found in "Inmate Gender," Federal Bureau of Prisons, accessed August 7, 2023, https://www.bop.gov/about /statistics/statistics_inmate_gender.jsp.

The quote from Nakeyda Haymer in chapter 8 is from Mallory Cheng, "Nakeyda Haymer Named Racine County's First Violent Crime Reduction Coordinator," WUWM, September 7, 2022, https:// www.wuwm.com/2022-09-07/nakeyda-haymer-is-named-racines -countys-first-violent-crime-reduction-coordinator. The quote from Mayor Jacob Frey is in Connor O'Neal, "Gun-Related Violence, Car- jackings Decrease during Minneapolis' 'Operation Endeavor,'" KARE 11 News, October 31, 2022, https://www.kare11.com/article/news /local/gun-related-violence-decrease-during-operation-endeavor /89-c1759f50-d650-4088-a77d-8fdd5f6ea141. The quote from Byron Brown is in Maki Becker, "Gun Violence Starts to Drop as Buffalo Po- lice Target Micro Hot Spots," *Buffalo News*, August 22, 2022, https:// buffalonews.com/news/local/crime-and-courts/gun-violence-starts -to-drop-as-buffalo-police-target-micro-hot-spots/article_fbcc4f30 -18d3-11ed-9b18-6b63d1ea647d.html#:~:text=%22This%20new%20 strategy%2C%20which%20is,on%20hot%20spots%20has%20critics. Information on the VICTIMS Act can be found at https://mcbath .house.gov/press-releases?ID=47E95C95-140D-43D0-B8EB-E8172 B70950D. The quote from Dr. Alexis R. Piquero is from a Department of Justice press release: "Department of Justice Awards More Than $26 Million to Support Criminal Justice Research and Statistics," US Department of Justice, Office of Justice Programs, November 2, 2022, https://www.ojp.gov/files/archives/pressreleases/2022/department -justice-awards-more-26-million-support-criminal-justice-research -and. The Thomas Abt quote about the Center for the Study and Practice of Violence Reduction is from "New Center Takes Aim at Rising Community Violence," *Maryland Today*, November 22, 2022, https://today.umd.edu/new-center-takes-aim-at-rising-community -violence.

INDEX